W9-BVC-257

Green Smoothies

FOR EVERY SEASON

A Year of Farmer's Market–Fresh Super Drinks

by **KRISTINE MILES**

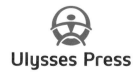

Ulysses Press

Published by
Ulysses Press
P.O. Box 3440
Berkeley, CA 94703
www.ulyssespress.com

ISBN: 978-1-61243-172-7
Library of Congress Catalog Number 2013931791

Printed in the United States by Bang Printing

10 9 8 7 6 5 4 3 2 1

Acquisitions editor: Keith Riegert
Editor: Lauren Harrison
Proofreader: Elyce Berrigan-Dunlop
Design: Jenna Stempel
Cover illustrations: front © Morphart Creation/shutterstock.com; back dandelion
   © Morphart Creation/shutterstock.com, strawberry leaves © Shlapak Liliya/shutterstock.com
Index: Sayre Van Young
Interior artwork: see page 128

Distributed by Publishers Group West

IMPORTANT NOTE TO READERS: This book is independently authored and published and no sponsorship or endorsement of this book by, and no affiliation with, any trademarked brands or other products mentioned or pictured within is claimed or suggested. All trademarks that appear in this book belong to their respective owners and are used here for informational purposes only. The author and publishers encourage readers to patronize the quality brands and products mentioned in this book.

To my dear parents and incredible husband,
who always support me and never doubt my ability to achieve anything.

Contents

Introduction

Smoothies come in many forms. Traditional smoothies are a combination of dairy milk or yogurt blended with ice and fruit, such as bananas or berries. Smoothies have also evolved to become supplemental delivery systems for protein powders and superfoods such as spirulina, maca, cacao, and acai berry. But what are green smoothies?

Green smoothies are smoothies with raw leafy greens blended through them. The emphasis is on leafy greens, not any green vegetable such as broccoli, peas, or zucchini. Traditionally, green smoothies are vegan, being a combination of sweet fruit, water, and leafy greens. However, green leaves can of course be blended through any type of smoothie, whether it is dairy- or plant-based. For the purposes of this book, green smoothie recipes have been designed without dairy products; some recipes include coconut water or nut milk.

There are many advantages to adding more greens to your diet, including the abundance of fiber, vitamins, minerals, and antioxidants, plus the alkaline value of raw greens and the benefits of blending rather than chewing.

If you have never had a green smoothie before, I can assure you that they taste a lot better than they look or sound. They do look green (and at times, other odd brown or purplish colors); however, they taste like the fruit in them. The ideal combination for 1 liter of green smoothie is 2 cups of fruit, 1½ cups of liquid, and 1 to 2 handfuls of leafy greens. This amount is perfect for two servings. The sweetness of the fruit offsets the flavor of what would otherwise be a bitter green drink. When using watery fruits like melons, recipes will use more fruit and little to no extra liquid.

To make a green smoothie, you put greens, coarsely chopped fruit, and liquid into a blender and blend for 1 to 2 minutes. Spinach is a great green for green smoothie beginners to start with as the flavor is mild and the color frequently spectacular. It is recommended to aim for 40 percent greens and 60 percent fruit. For beginners, start with a small amount of greens and gradually increase over time to 40 percent greens—or more. If you do happen to overdo the greens, try adding some sweetener, a bit of vanilla extract, or some lemon juice to take the edge off.

Specific greens are suggested for each recipe in this book taking into account variety, the season, and flavor matching. Should you not have the suggested green available, of course feel free to substitute it for something else. The amount of green is also up to you. For beginners, start with a small handful and build up as tolerated. For experienced green smoothie drinkers, you will know how much you like to use. The amount of leafy green suggested takes into account how strong the green is; however, this can vary worldwide. For instance I understand romaine lettuce has a stronger flavor in Australia than it does in the U.S.

For those with underactive thyroid issues who wish to avoid raw goitrogenic greens, substitute as necessary. Leafy greens considered goitrogenic include bok choy, cabbage, collards, watercress, kale, radish tops, turnip greens, and, to a lesser extent, spinach.

Sweeteners are suggested for some recipes to compensate for the use of semisweet and sour fruits. Feel free to replace the suggested sweetener (usually dates, honey, or agave) with an alternative should you prefer one, like coconut nectar or stevia. See page 30 for more info on natural sweeteners.

Suggestions for use of almond or other nut milks, or coconut water, are for texture, flavor, or nutrient profiles. Should they not be available, or not preferred, use plain water or whatever liquid you are comfortable with. See page 35 for how easy it is to make homemade almond milk.

For regular green smoothie consumers, a high-powered blender is highly recommended, such as Vitamix or Blendtec brands. My preferred brand is Thermomix, which is a multifunction appliance that includes a high-powered blender function. It is readily available in the UK, Europe, and Australia. Less expensive blenders still work, but you may need to rest the motor if its gets warm with the effort of blending the greens for a couple of minutes, and it will break down quickly with very regular use.

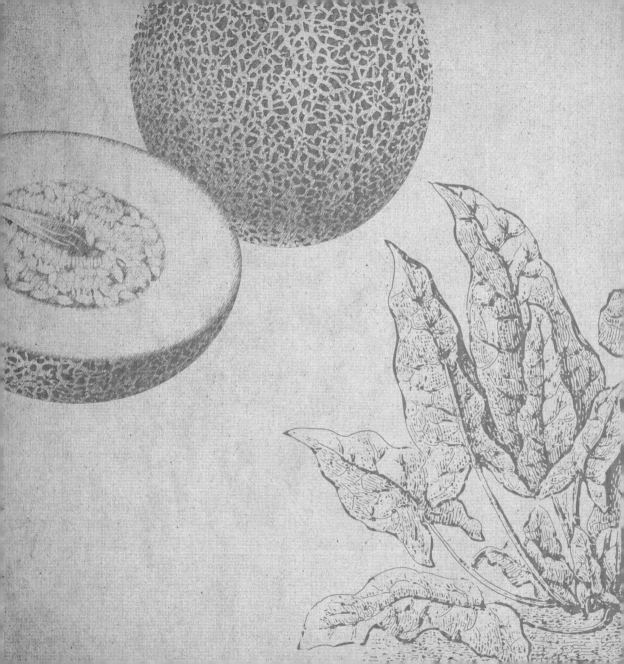

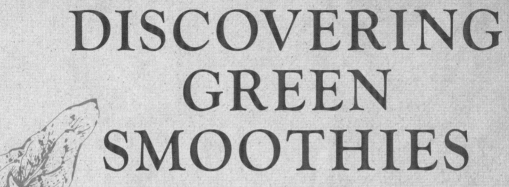

DISCOVERING GREEN SMOOTHIES

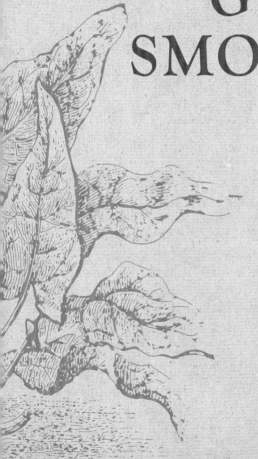

Green Smoothie Inspiration

My inspiration to drink green smoothies came from reading *Green for Life* by Victoria Boutenko in 2007. I have had a green smoothie for breakfast almost every day since, which is well over 1,500 smoothies! My passion for the humble green drink and knowledge of the human body resulted in the creation of my own blog in 2008, and subsequently my first book, *The Green Smoothie Bible*, published in 2012.

The reason I love green smoothies and continue to drink them for breakfast is they see me through all the way to lunchtime and they are just so convenient. The combination of fiber, fruit-based carbohydrates, and an abundance of nutrients from the fruit and greens results in stable blood sugar and I am satisfied. I can also blend my smoothie quickly, and if there's no time to drink it at home, it goes in a glass jar and I take it to work with me. Whenever I have a more "traditional" breakfast, I don't feel the same. If I only eat fruit or have a juice, I need to eat a couple of hours later, or if I have something grain- or nut-based, I just feel heavy in the guts and sluggish.

I am a once-a-day, half-a-liter green smoothie drinker. I know others that drink 1 to 1½ liters daily and others that just have one occasionally. Whether you drink a lot or a little, green smoothies are beneficial to your health. You don't need to be raw vegan to enjoy green smoothies, and you don't have to drink them every day, but the more blended greens you can get into your diet, the better.

Here are some testimonials from people who have introduced green smoothies into their diets:

"Armed with my morning green smoothie, I have energy all day. In my 60th year I swam the Channel Challenge and Phillip Island Swim Classic, walked the Oxfam 100km walk in 37 hours, spent my 60th birthday riding a horse across the Steppe in Mongolia, and walked the Kokoda Track. I am a pretty good advertisement for green smoothies, I reckon!"
    —JULIE T., VICTORIA, AUSTRALIA

"I started making green smoothies for my breakfast as a desperate attempt to increase my fruit and greens intake. I'd read about the health benefits of having more greens in my diet, but as a working mum, I didn't have the time to make different meals. After my first green smoothie I was converted. It was easy to prepare, tasted great, and filled me up. I've since noticed my energy rise, skin condition improve, and my fruit and greens intake significantly increase."
    —CLAIRE H., SUSSEX, UK

"Optimum health was extremely important to my husband and me while we were trying to conceive. We wanted our bodies to be as healthy as possible, and also ensure we gave our baby the healthiest start too. Green smoothies made that so easy! We had such fun seeing what new and delicious combinations we could come up with. We have so much energy, our skin is amazing, we have a healthy baby on the way, and we really love that it is a quick, easy way to get a lot of nutrients into our systems."
    —STEPHANIE S., WESTERN AUSTRALIA, AUSTRALIA

"I knew quickly that green smoothies were the tastiest and most efficient way to fast-track my optimum health. Results were immediate and many years later, my love affair with blended greens is still going strong! Green smoothies enhance my digestion (from all that soothing and filling fiber), and they help me stay satisfied and alkalized on a high-raw, vegan diet. Following a presentation by edible weeds expert Sergei Boutenko, I gained confidence to add nutrition-dense weeds such as plantain, nettle, and purslane to my smoothies. If you change nothing else about your diet, I urge you to add in green smoothies and watch the magic happen!"
  —LUCY S., VICTORIA, AUSTRALIA

"I discovered green smoothies between my first and second babies about eight months ago. I attribute my energy (despite sleep deprivation), health (no coughs, colds, or illnesses in general), and excellent recovery from another gruelling birth to this amazing drink. It's cheap (especially when you can grow some of your own greens), easy, delicious, and filling. I feel clean from the inside out. My husband and I now can't go a day without that feeling of inner cleanliness and vitality that comes from 'green goodness.'"
  —LAURA S., QUEENSLAND, AUSTRALIA

Health Benefits

FIBER

Most people do not consume the 25 to 30 grams of fiber recommended daily, and the incidence of high cholesterol, type 2 diabetes, constipation, and bowel cancer are huge in Western countries. Increasing fiber is recommended for all of these conditions for prevention and treatment, and green smoothies are an excellent way of getting more fiber into your diet. Smoothies are easy on the digestive process like juices are, but have the advantage of retaining the fiber, not eliminating it. Green smoothies are fiber rich by nature because of the greens *and* fruit content.

There are two types of fiber. Insoluble fiber is largely from the greens and is the "roughage" that acts like a broom to sweep our colons clean and helps maintain intestinal pH, which is the balance between acid and alkaline. Soluble fiber breaks down into much smaller pieces, forming a gel that helps form our stools, making them easier to pass. Soluble fiber is also important as it assists with blood sugar regulation by slowing the release of glucose into the bloodstream, and it aids the removal of low-density lipoprotein ("bad" cholesterol) from the body via the bowel. Fruits rich in soluble fiber are most ideal, as their action is gentler on the digestive tract. Such fruits include apples, bananas, blueberries, citrus, kiwifruit, mangoes, pears, plums, and strawberries. Extra fiber-rich additions to smoothies can include chia seeds, beets, and oats.

BLENDING GREENS

Nutrients are stored within a plant's cells, and their cell walls (made of hardy cellulose) need to be ruptured to release them. Unfortunately, humans don't have the jaw strength or the time to chew on greens till they are a creamy consistency like apes do. Blending or juicing greens ruptures cells with ease, making nutrients more readily available, and effectively predigests the plants involved. The key difference is that the fiber is retained when blending, which is a good thing. Moreover, the use of raw greens means that all nutrients are available, unlike the loss of vitamins and the denaturing of protein that occurs with cooking.

Green smoothies are frequently consumed for breakfast, a time where greens rarely make an appearance. Hence blending greens in a smoothie for breakfast is another way to get more greens into your diet as a whole. A green smoothie is also a lot more convenient to prepare than a green juice. The preparation and cleanup of a smoothie takes a matter of minutes, compared to the time-consuming process of juicing and the very messy clean-up afterward.

ANTIOXIDANTS

Oxidation, degradation, rusting—these are all terms to describe the breakdown of a substance due to a chemical reaction with its surroundings. The classic example is the rusting of iron into iron oxide by exposure to water. Degradation due to "oxidation" occurs not only on metals, but in the human body too.

If not balanced, oxidizing reactions lead to the formation of "free radicals," which can lead to cellular damage if they are not neutralized by "antioxidants." Free radical formation in the human body can be affected by tobacco smoke, toxins, pollution, stress, and poor eating habits. It is believed that free radical damage can accelerate the progression of cancer, cardiovascular disease, rheumatoid arthritis, chronic fatigue, and age-related diseases. Hence a diet rich in antioxidants, which exist in plants and algae, makes for the ideal army to fight the existence of free radicals.

Examples of antioxidant substances are vitamins A, C, and E, the mineral selenium, coenzyme Q10, glutathione, flavonoids, polyphenols, and pigments that color plants, such as chlorophyll and carotenoids. Berries, brightly colored fruits, herbs, spices, and dark and red-green leaves have the highest antioxidant powers in the plant kingdom.

The antioxidant pigment chlorophyll is what makes green leaves "green." It is based on a magnesium ion and is similar in structure to hemoglobin, the red pigment in our red blood cells based on iron. Not only is chlorophyll an antioxidant, it is anti-inflammatory, detoxifying, and promotes healing, making it extremely beneficial for the human body.

MINERALS

Leafy greens are a very nutrient-dense food. Naturally, different greens have different nutrient profiles, but if you eat a variety of them, you will consume an abundance of minerals, namely potassium, magnesium, calcium, iron, zinc, manganese, sodium, sulphur, and selenium!

Calcium	This mineral what makes up our skeleton, and like magnesium, it is important for our nerves and muscles. Vitamin D assists with the absorption of calcium.
Iron	Iron's primary role is to transport oxygen in our blood, forming the center of each hemoglobin molecule. Non-heme iron from plants requires vitamin C to aid its absorption.
Magnesium	Magnesium is used by every organ in the body and contributes to the health of our teeth and bones in partnership with calcium. An important mineral for relaxation, magnesium may assist with muscle tension, restless legs, fibromyalgia, and nervous disorders.

Manganese	Manganese is essential to facilitate a multitude of enzyme reactions in the body. It is also necessary to aid absorption of vitamins C and B, and supports a healthy thyroid.
Potassium	Potassium is an important electrolyte mineral, playing a key role in muscle contraction and nerve transmission, including its role in lowering risk of high blood pressure.
Selenium	Selenium is an antioxidant mineral that fights free radicals; it may play an important role in preventing cancer. It is also essential for underactive thyroid conditions.
Zinc	Zinc is very important for our immune function, wound healing, and DNA and protein synthesis. It is vitally important for the growth and development of babies, children, and teenagers.

VITAMINS

Like the abundance of minerals in leafy greens, vitamins A, C, E, and K, and B-group vitamins are well represented and essential to the human body for excellent health and well-being.

Vitamin A	Vitamin A is an antioxidant vitamin critical for the health of our eyes. It is also very important for thyroid function and for the maintenance of our major organs, such as our heart and kidneys.
Vitamins B1, B2, and B3	Vitamins B1, B2, and B3 assist the body in producing energy. They also influence enzyme reactions that help to regulate the function of our muscles, nerves, and heart.
Vitamin B5	Vitamin B5 is involved with hormone regulation and supports the adrenal gland, assisting with glowing healthy skin and stress management.

Vitamin B6	Vitamin B6 is important for the health of red blood cells, as well as our immune and nervous systems. It also assists with protein metabolism and blood sugar regulation.
Folate	Folate is a B vitamin essential for the neurological development of a growing baby and the reproduction of DNA in our cells, and is very important for our mood.
Vitamin C	Vitamin C is important for our immune system due to its powerful antioxidant properties. Its role in collagen formation makes it essential for soft tissue healing.
Vitamin K	Vitamin K is abundant in many greens and plays numerous important roles in the body, particularly the regulation of blood clotting. Additionally, vitamin K protects against diabetes, heart disease, cancer, osteoporosis, Alzheimer's, and arthritis.

ALKALINITY

pH is a measure of whether a substance is acid or alkaline. If pH is below 7, it's acidic; 7 is neutral, and above 7 is alkaline. Human blood needs to be between a pH of 7.35 to 7.45, which means it is slightly alkaline. It is a constant balancing act for the body to keep the blood within this range with different nutrients. The action of breathing is the main regulator of blood pH due to the exchange of oxygen and carbon dioxide; however, minerals are also used, such as calcium to increase pH and phosphorous to reduce pH.

Negative attitudes and behaviors, toxins, and certain foods are considered "acid-forming," and the opposite are "alkaline-forming." Acid- or alkaline-forming is the effect at a blood and cellular level, versus how something tastes. For example, lemon juice tastes acidic, but is alkaline-forming to the blood. Alcohol, sugar, grains, roasted nuts, animal products, junk foods, and fried fats are all acid-forming to the body. When such foods form the majority of the diet, the body must work very hard to "alkalize" to find balance, drawing precious minerals like calcium and magnesium from our bones in the process.

Raw fruits, vegetables, plant-based raw fats such as coconut and avocado, and *especially leafy greens* are naturally alkalizing to the body. Eating a diet that is around 70 percent alkaline means minerals are not depleted and the body can use its energy for healing and growth rather than for reducing acidity.

ROTATING YOUR GREENS

Eating seasonally is what this book is all about, and it makes sense to eat what is growing now, eating what nature intended us to eat at certain times of the year. Eating according to the seasons will also ensure you eat different greens, which is important for the following two reasons.

There are naturally occurring substances in plants called "secondary metabolites"; for example, chard and spinach have oxalic acid in them, herbs have essential oils, and some greens have tannins, nitrates, phytates, or saponins. If you eat the same green in your smoothie every day, you may start to have problems with too many of the same metabolites in your system, which is harmless in small quantities, but can be dangerous or unpleasant in large amounts. The point of these naturally occurring substances in plants is that they make us rotate our food sources. In the wild, this is a defense mechanism to prevent devastation by predators. I can tell if I have been eating too much of the same green because I start to not want green smoothies and I feel a bit queasy midmorning.

The impact of this plant defense mechanism in a modern society (where we are not foraging wild animals) is to be sure we eat a variety of foods, which is important nutritionally. Eating a wide variety of greens will ensure we get the broad spectrum of vitamins, minerals, and antioxidants available across the plant kingdom.

GROWING WITH THE SEASON

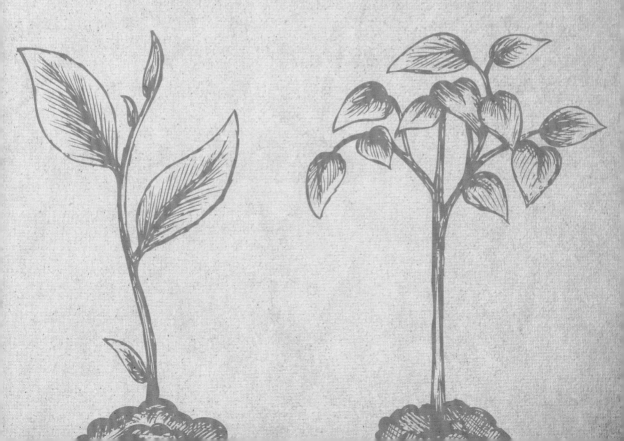

Sourcing Fresh Fruit and Greens

There is no doubt that "fresh is best," and short of growing your own fruit and vegetables, the next best thing is to buy from farmers markets, where the grower directly sells their produce. Even if the farmer is not selling certified-organic produce, they can tell you if their methods are chemical-free or not, and commonly their goods have been picked just the day before. Farmers markets are often much cheaper than commercial stores, especially if you buy in bulk. Almost all stallholders will happily "do a deal" for a whole box of something at a reduced price, particularly toward the end of the market when they are hoping to sell out of their stock on hand.

While "certified-organic" is a guarantee your food is chemical-free and not genetically modified, even organic produce in a supermarket can be doubted for its freshness factor, with nutrition losses as storage and shelf time lengthens. The most important thing, however, is to do the very best you can with the resources you have available. For taste and nutrition, it's best if you can get chemical-free produce from a farmers market, or you can grow your own. If all you have is a produce department in a supermarket, then this is still better than nothing at all. Just be sure to wash the fresh greens and fruits in plenty of water with a splash of apple cider vinegar to eliminate pesticide residues.

Sticking to a whole-food way of eating takes planning. Having multiple places to source fresh produce is the best way to ensure you always have a full fruit bowl and a stocked fridge. Personally, I don't just rely on my local farmers market because it only happens once a month. I am also part of a co-op, where I can order a mixed fruit and vegetable box weekly.

I grow herbs and greens in pots on my porch, and my mother supplies me with seasonal greens from her garden. I also stock up at the supermarket as needed.

You can consider all of these options for sourcing fresh produce:

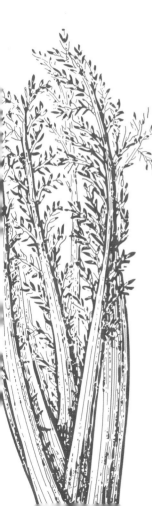

- Grow your own

- Barter excess produce you have grown with other growers (such as neighbors)

- Make good friends with people who grow too much and are generous!

- Join a community garden

- Join or create a co-op

- Visit farmers markets

- Source more obscure ingredients from Asian markets and grocery stores

- Look out for health food or whole-food stores selling organic produce

- Purchase organic or conventional produce from a supermarket

Ripeness Is in the Variety

Planning on planting a couple of fruit trees in your garden? Maybe a nice little orchard? Add variety for a year filled with ripe fruit! Of course, if you don't have room to grow your own fruits and vegetables, there tends to be some variety of your favorite fruit that's just about to ripen at any given time during the year.

That's because not all varieties of a fruit are ready for harvest at the same time. For example, while apples are typically widely available from July all the way up to December, specific types of apple have their own specific season of harvest; Yellow Transparents will begin showing up starting as early as mid-June, while you won't find Pink Ladies at their ripest until mid-October. The same is true for everything from berries and melons to stone fruit. For example Desert Delight nectarines are best at summer solstice where as Liz's Late nectarines are ready at the end of August.

And while growing seasons vary widely depending on latitude and climate (or hemisphere), the basic fruits chart on page 25 will give you a good selection of "fall back fruits," fruits where at least one varietal will be ripe and at their nutrient-packed best at any given time of the year.

For specific harvesting information, especially when it comes to local farmers markets, I highly recommend doing some research online, where you can find harvest charts from local farms and orchards.

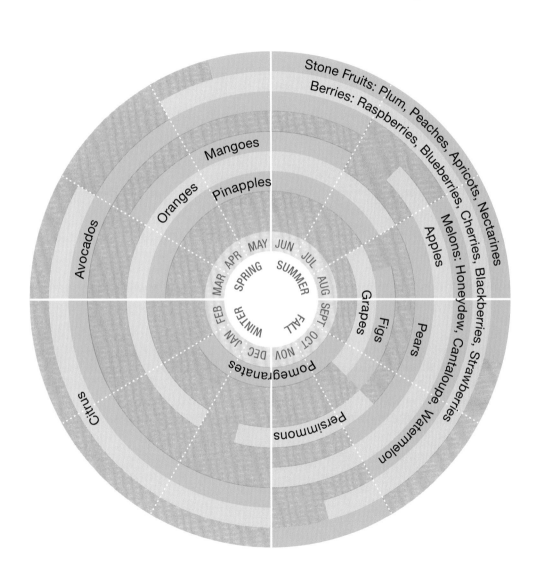

Stone Fruits: Plum, Peaches, Apricots, Nectarines
Berries: Raspberries, Blueberries, Cherries, Blackberries, Strawberries
Melons: Honeydew, Cantaloupe, Watermelon
Mangoes
Oranges
Pinapples
Avocados
Apples
Grapes
Figs
Pears
Citrus
Pomegranates
Persimmons

SPRING
SUMMER
FALL
WINTER

MAR APR MAY JUN JUL AUG SEPT OCT NOV DEC JAN FEB

An Abundance of Green

Like fruits, each type of green you harvest from your garden or find fresh at the farmer's market has its own peak season. While opportunities to enjoy your favorite greens at their freshest and most nutritious come and go often far too quickly, pay attention and you're sure to find a new favorite green at almost any time during the year. Beet greens often shoot up before any other green appears in the early spring garden, where as kale is at its most delectable and healthy all the way up to the new year.

Growing your own greens for the freshest smoothies possible? Two of the best pieces of gardening advice I've ever received were the following:

1. Pick your greens early in the morning (the perfect time for a morning smoothie!) when, as the plant prepares for the growing day, sap rises up the leaves giving them a nutritious and flavorful boost.

2. Freeze what you can't eat. Like fruit, the nutritional power of leafy greens diminishes quickly the further out from harvesting they get. Combine that with relatively short harvest months and you may find yourself with a bushel of kale about to go to waste. Instead, lock in the nutrients and save everything for later by freezing what you won't use now. To save freezer space, puree the greens and freeze in ice cube trays. Once frozen, pop the green cubes in a sealed container or bag.

For a quick glance of some common greens you'll find throughout the year, see the basic greens chart on page 27.

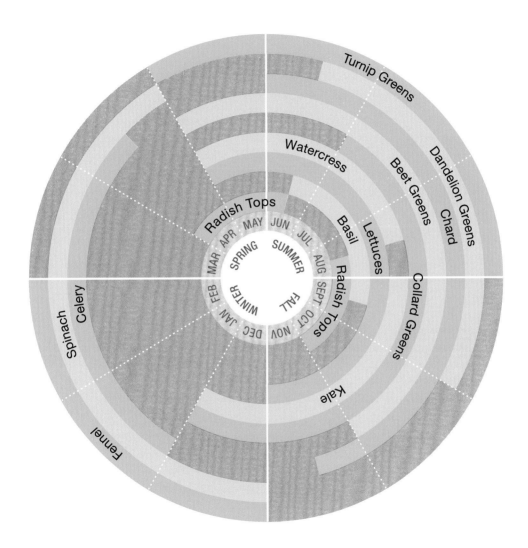

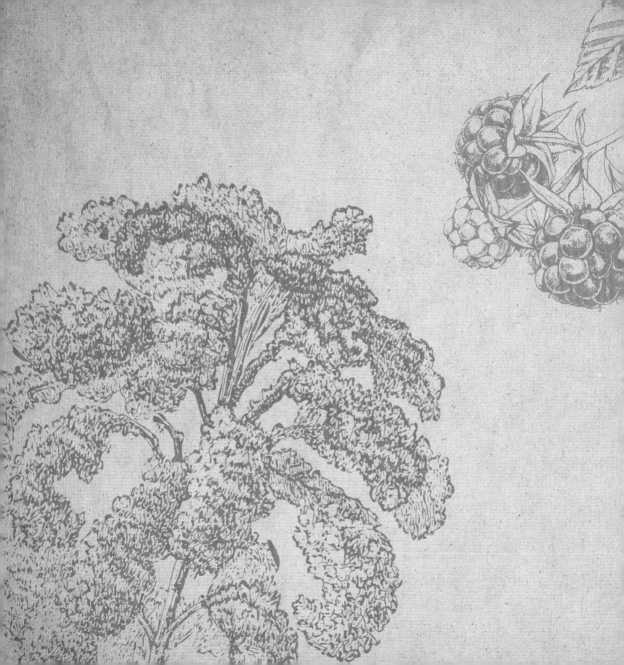

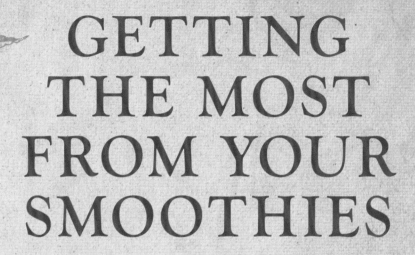

GETTING THE MOST FROM YOUR SMOOTHIES

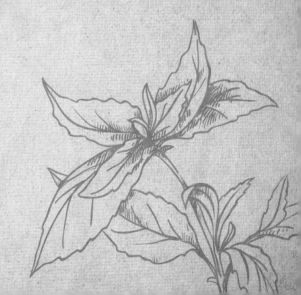

Natural Sweeteners

To make a green smoothie delicious, it is necessary to balance bitterness and sourness with sweetness. Ideally, the fruit supplies this sweet flavor, but sometimes it's not enough. Natural sweeteners used sparingly are the solution.

Honey
The best choice is unheated and unfiltered honey, full of nutrients such as enzymes, B vitamins, minerals, pollens, and propolis. Regular consumption of raw honey from your local area is thought to assist with controlling seasonal allergies.

Agave nectar
Extracted from the Mexican agave cactus, this sweet and inulin-rich syrup is high in fructose, making it low GI. Inulin is a fructan that has beneficial effects on gut flora, but is not suited to those with fructose/fructan malabsorption.

Dried fruits
Dates, raisins, and golden raisins are concentrated sources of fruity sweetness. Try soaking them overnight, making them easier to blend. Soft Medjool dates are the best option, as they're rich in iron, potassium, calcium, manganese, and vitamin B6.

Coconut sugar
This caramel-flavored sugar has a low GI of 35, is an incredibly sustainable crop to grow, and is a source of iron, magnesium, and zinc. It's widely available in granulated forms; also look out for the delicious coconut nectar that the sugar is made from.

Stevia
With leaves 250 times sweeter than sugar and zero calories, stevia is the best option for avoiding processed or unprocessed forms of sugar. Available in leaf, powder, or tablet forms, stevia doesn't taste as pleasant as other natural sweeteners.

Herbs

Tender, fragrant herbs are fabulous additions to green smoothies. They add flavor and deliver an abundance of nutrition and medicinal benefits. The four most commonly available and most useful herbs in green smoothies are basil, mint, cilantro, and parsley.

Herbs contain volatile essential oils and antioxidant vitamins, flavonoids, and pigments, and these four herbs have all similar properties, including the ability to calm a stressed or anxious nervous system, yet energize a system that requires stimulation. All four are digestive aids, are antibacterial and anti-inflammatory, and possess anticancer properties. They all contain, to varying degrees, vitamins C, A, and K, as well as folate, iron, manganese, and calcium.

Basil   The aroma of basil is good for memory and concentration, particularly in times of mental fatigue. Basil is particularly rich in vitamin K. It also contains zeathanthin, a carotenoid antioxidant that protects the eye. Basil is warming and can have a clovelike taste. In green smoothies, basil goes well with cilantro, coconut milk, fig, ginger, lemon, lime, mint, and tomato.

Mint   Varieties of mint include spearmint, apple mint, pineapple mint, peppermint, and even chocolate mint. In addition to a broad spectrum of vitamins and minerals, mint also contains omega-3 oils, vitamin E, vitamin B2, potassium, and magnesium. In green smoothies, mint goes well with basil, cilantro, citrus, cucumber, ginger, kiwifruit, lemon, lime, melon, parsley, pineapple, and tomato.

Cilantro   The leaves of this medicinal herb are known as cilantro in the United States and Latin America, and the seeds are known as coriander. In Asia, Australia, and the United Kingdom the leaves and seeds are both referred to as coriander. Cilantro is considered a good herb for diabetics as it helps to regulate insulin activity. It also helps lower cholesterol by improving the digestion of fat. In green smoothies, cilantro goes well with avocado, basil, beets, coconut, cucumber, ginger, kiwifruit, lemon, lime, mint, parsley, and pineapple.

Parsley   High amounts of vitamin C and iron make parsley an excellent source of iron for vegetarians, because non-heme iron from plants is harder for the body to absorb than heme iron found in animal foods, and vitamin C increases the uptake of iron in the body. Parsley also contains all of the B vitamins and is excellent for detoxification due to its very high antioxidant content. In green smoothies, parsley goes well with avocado, cabbage, cardamom, cilantro, citrus, cucumber, kale, kumquat, lemon, mint, and pomegranate.

Microgreens and Sprouts

Sprouts are germinated seeds with a young root stem, with either two or no leaves, and are eaten whole. Examples are alfalfa, lentil, and mung. Microgreens are little seedlings. They have larger stems than sprouts and clear leaf development. They are harvested by cutting the stem off the root. Examples are cress and sunflower shoots. Basil, beet, and cilantro microgreens are also delicious and frequently used as culinary garnishes.

Both sprouts and microgreens are little powerhouses of nutrition and flavor, and super-fun to grow at home at any time of year. Sprouts are best grown in a glass jar covered with hosiery or tulle, and fastened with an elastic band. Soak seeds overnight then drain and rinse well. Rinse twice daily and drain on a 45-degree angle away from direct sunlight till ready (three to seven days). Sprouts will stay fresh in the fridge for a few days.

Microgreens are grown on soil or porous stones and gently watered like regular plants. They are germinated in the dark, and grown in indirect sunlight for one to three weeks, either indoors near a window or in a covered outdoor porch area. Harvest and use immediately as needed.

Both sprouts and microgreens can have a strong flavor, so for use in green smoothies, they are best used in combination with another mild, larger green such as spinach or Swiss chard.

Nuts and Seeds

Little powerhouses of minerals, protein, fiber, and healthy fats, nuts and seeds are excellent additions to green smoothies. They can be used to add bulk to a smoothie to make it more filling and can also add creaminess. They are helpful for adding specific nutrients such as calcium from almonds, zinc from sunflower and pumpkin seeds, magnesium from cashews, selenium from Brazil nuts, or omega-3 fats from hemp seeds, walnuts, or chia seeds. Fats are also necessary to aid the absorption of minerals and fat-soluble vitamins such as A, D, E, and K.

Milks	Homemade nut and seed milks are simple to make and can be used as a substitute for water in any recipe. See page 35 on how to make your own nut and seed milks.
Butters	Ground nuts or seeds, either made at home in a high-speed blender or bought commercially, can be used to create a quick milk. Simply use 1 tablespoon per cup of water added to your smoothie.
Whole nuts and seeds	Add approximately 2 tablespoons of nuts or seeds per cup of water, and this will create a similar consistency to adding a nut or seed butter. To aid digestion, soak the nuts or seeds overnight and discard the soaking water before adding to the smoothie. Hemp seeds do not need soaking.
Chia seeds	Chia can be presoaked or added dry to a smoothie. The latter will result in the smoothie getting considerably thicker.

NUT AND SEED MILKS

To make homemade milk, first you need to soak your nut or seed of choice. Soaking helps to deactivate substances that are stopping the nut or seed from growing, particularly protease inhibitors (protease is an enzyme that helps break down protein). Soaking also aids the removal of antinutrients like phytates, which can interfere with mineral absorption. The addition of salt to the soak water helps with the removal of these substances. Eating nuts and seeds after they have been soaked is more kind to our digestion and improves nutrient availability.

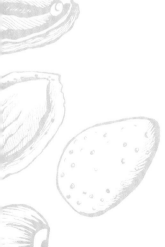

- Soak macadamias, cashews, pistachios, and pine nuts for 2 to 4 hours in filtered or spring water.

- Soak almonds, Brazil nuts, hazelnuts, sunflower seeds, pumpkin seeds (pepitas), sesame seeds, pistachios, pecans, or walnuts overnight or all day.

- Add ½ teaspoon salt to the soaking water per cup of nuts or seeds.

- Once soaked, drain and rinse the nuts or seeds very well.

- Combine the soaked nuts or seeds (1 cup dry weight) to 4½ cups of water, and blend for 1 minute on high speed.

- Strain the mixture though a nut milk bag or fine cloth set over a large bowl. You will need to massage the liquid out of the fiber; it's messy but good fun! You can use the leftover fiber in other recipes to save wastage, or try it as a face and body scrub.

- Store the milk in the fridge and use within 3 days. This recipe is perfect for making 3 (1-liter) green smoothies, per the recipes in this book.

Coconuts

Coconut oil is a saturated fat, which refers to its structure having all its possible links filled with hydrogen atoms. Unlike the long-chain saturated fats from animal products, coconut oil is a medium-chain fat. Because it is shorter, it is metabolized by the body quickly and efficiently into energy. Given it raises our metabolism, it can aid weight loss. Moreover, in contrast to saturated animal fat, coconut oil helps to raise our good HDL cholesterol levels.

Coconut is 47 percent lauric acid, which is the fat in breast milk that makes it so special. Fresh coconut milk is so rich in electrolytes such as potassium that it was used in old war times as an emergency replacement for blood plasma. Combined with magnesium-rich greens in green smoothies, coconut water is a match made in nutrition heaven for blood health!

Coconut aids digestion, is good for blood sugar, aids absorption of minerals and fat-soluble vitamins, and is antifungal, antiviral, and antibacterial, hence it's great for the immune system. Coconut also nourishes the thyroid and supports cardiovascular health.

The flesh and water from young coconuts are well-suited to green smoothies. The flesh is soft and imparts a lovely, silky texture. Coconut water is delicately sweet. Coconut oil can be added to smoothies also, but will need to be soft or runny so it blends well. At less than 65°F (18°C), coconut oil becomes hard, and above 79°F (26°C), it will turn to liquid.

HOW TO OPEN A COCONUT

The coconuts referred to in this book are young or green coconuts, sometimes called drinking coconuts. They look cylindrical and white with a pointed top and a flat bottom. Over the years I have gone from a method of opening them that was very messy, with bits of husk and liquid flying everywhere, to one that is very safe and simple!

- Turn the coconut on its side. With a large knife, shave the white husk off the pointed end down to the pale brown shell.

- Turn the coconut up onto its base again. On the top there are three thick lines that meet at the apex. With the heel of the same knife, tap firmly on one of these lines about halfway along until it cracks the shell; not much force is needed.

- Stick the heel of the knife in the crack, and with a bit of leverage, you will create a continuation of the crack in a perfect circle around the top that you can prise open.

- Empty the water into a bowl through a fine-mesh sieve to catch any debris, and check that the water is a clear/white color. If it's pink, purple, or brown, or it doesn't taste amazing, throw it out!

- To scoop out the flesh, use the back of a soup spoon to peel the flesh off the shell. You should almost be able to remove it in one piece if it's thick enough. Rinse under water and scrape off any brown bits from the shell.

Protein

Protein has become a bit of a buzz word in recent years, and with so much emphasis on "consuming enough protein" you would think we are in danger of becoming deficient. As long as you eat a nutritious and balanced diet, there is no danger of protein deficiency.

Carbohydrates are what we primarily need for energy, fat is what we primarily need for our brain and endocrine systems, and protein is essential for growth and repair. The most rapid period of growth in our lives is our first six months. Breast milk is the perfect food for an infant and contains 6 percent of its calories from protein. The World Health Organization recommends we consume only 10 percent of our calories from protein to ensure we do get the 5 to 6 percent we actually need.

It is important to eat protein at each meal if you wish to lose weight and keep your blood sugar levels even; however, this doesn't mean you should eat a slab of meat at every sitting. There is an abundance of protein-rich plants, and this includes green leaves! You'll also get protein from seed grains like quinoa, chia, and amaranth, and nuts, seeds, legumes, and sprouts such as alfalfa.

Green smoothies are a great source of protein when you are consuming a good 40 percent of your smoothie as greens. Spinach has 30 percent of its calories as protein compared to cheese at 26 percent and beef at 50 percent. Given that cooking destroys protein by 50 percent, 4 ounces (100 grams) of cooked beef is similar to around 3.5 ounces (80 grams) of raw spinach for available protein content.

Cleansing

A "cleanse" or a "detox" can come in many forms. Some authorities say our bodies don't need to be detoxed by any particular program because our bodies are in a constant state of detoxification via the function of the liver in particular. This is true, but we live in a toxic world and many diets are not ideal. As a result, the world is full of chronic illness and disease.

Ask anyone who has performed a cleanse, and they know it has an effect. For some, it isn't pleasant, as they release toxins too quickly and go through what is known as a "healing crisis," which is temporary but can include flulike symptoms.

Increasing in popularity are liquid cleanses using juices or smoothies or both for one day or multiple days. For juice cleanses (or juice fasts or feasts), you need to make a lot of juice because they go through your system so quickly. Unless they are made for you, it can be a messy and time-consuming process.

Cleansing using green smoothies is an alternative, and due to the fiber, most people find 2 liters of smoothie spread over three to four meals very satisfying. You can choose to drink all sweet fruit smoothies, or you may prefer to have a savory green smoothie at dinnertime. There is one savory recipe per season in this book and a larger selection in *The Green Smoothie Bible*.

SPRINGING INTO SPRING

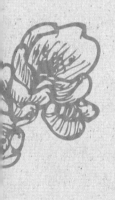

After a harsh, cold winter, spring is such a beautiful and welcome time of year. Flowers bloom and everyone starts to smile more as the sun shines brightly and begins to warm our world. Spring is, however, a surprisingly limited time for produce, as gardens are just being planted for later harvests.

Fruits available in early spring are largely left over from winter and include citruses like grapefruits and kumquats. The beautiful blood oranges, grown in sunny areas and only around for a short time in late winter and early spring, are not to be missed.

Late spring heralds the start of fruits that lead us into summer and include bananas, raspberries, strawberries, melons, and tropical fruits like lychees and mangoes. After many months of eating predominantly citrus, apples, and pears, it is utterly delightful to relish that first strawberry of the season, with its succulent, sweet flesh. The magical taste of those first few fresh berries (that haven't been transported halfway around the world) is such a welcome return.

In contrast to spring fruits, seasonal greens are more abundant as everything green is racing to grow. Year-round staples like Swiss chard, endive, and radish tops are still producing, while herbs, lettuce varieties, beet greens, and cabbages become plentiful. Tender pea shoots and watercress are extraordinary spring superfoods.

SPRING FRUITS

While early spring fruits can be limited to leftover winter citrus, avocados and the green smoothie staple, bananas, are at their best.

Avocados   Avocados are rich in healthy monounsaturated fats and vitamins C, E, and folate, as well as green, orange, *and* yellow antioxidant pigments. The presence of good-quality fats is important for the assimilation of fat-soluble nutrients such as vitamins A, C, and D, and carotenoid pigments. Avocados are also great additions to green smoothies for added creaminess and thickness.

Bananas   Bananas are the best fruit source of vitamin B6, which helps with the production of neurotransmitters important for mood. Bananas also contain heart-healthy potassium, vitamin C, and other B group vitamins. Despite its "high-carb" label in the world of high-protein diets, bananas have an average low GI score of 52, making them a very healthy snack and staple green smoothie ingredient that is available all year round.

Kumquats   Kumquats, tart and delectable, are considered by farmers and botanists alike to be members of the citrus family, but they aren't. Officially, this incredible little fruit gets its own genus—Fortunella. Regardless of what you call them, kumquats make an excellent, powerfully flavorful addition to your smoothies with high levels of flavanoid antioxidants and vitamin C to complement the sweet and sour taste. The best part? Unlike citrus fruits that have to be cut and peeled, you can toss in kumquats whole!

SPRING FRUITS FROM THE TROPICS

Without a lot of regional fruits in season, spring is a fantastic time to throw some tropical flavor into your green smoothies. Most large grocery stores and some farmers markets carry organic varieties, or you can always opt for fresh-frozen packs, which help keep the fruits' nutrients from degrading.

Mangoes Mangoes are considered the "symbol of love" in India and worldwide are known as the "king of fruit." Available in late spring and summer, this stone fruit has more antioxidant beta-carotene than any other fruit. It is also a source of vitamin C, potassium, and calcium, is rich in soluble fiber, and due to its enzyme properties (similar to papaya), it is well known as a digestive aid.

Papayas Ancient Mayans worshipped papaya trees, calling them the "tree of life," which is understandable given they contain vitamins A, C, and E, and B vitamins, potassium, and antioxidants such as beta-carotene and lutein, which are important for eye health. While you can get papaya all year round, they are more readily available in winter and spring. Papaya, particularly when unripe, contains papain, an enzyme that helps digest protein. It is used in cooking to tenderize meat and can be used to aid digestion.

Pineapples Available year round, pineapples are best in late spring and early summer. They don't ripen or get sweeter and softer once picked but will get juicier after harvesting. Pineapple is rich in vitamins A and C, as well as anti-inflammatory antioxidants such as bromelain, which is also a protein-digesting enzyme. This fruit is an excellent source of manganese, a mineral essential to many bodily processes, including the processing of cholesterol, protein, and carbs, for blood sugar maintenance, thyroid health, and it aids the absorption of vitamins B and C.

SPRING GREENS

Winter is full of robust greens like celery, fennel, and kale to match our diet, which requires more dense foods for satiety in the cooler months. Then along comes spring, with greens that are light and tender, such as the myriad of lettuce varieties that are perfect for crisp salads and spring green smoothies.

Cabbage Cabbage is part of the large brassica family alongside kale, bok choy, collards, turnip greens, and watercress. Cabbage possesses, as all the brassicas do, a plentiful supply of glucosinolates, which convert to isothiocyanates (ITCs). ITCs such as sulforaphane and indole-3-carbinol (I3C) are known to be protective against breast, prostate, and colon cancers, are anti-inflammatory, and can help to heal stomach ulcers due to the helicobacter pylori infection. Cabbage itself is an excellent source of vitamins C and K, and a very good source of folate and manganese.

Lettuce Lettuce comes in countless varieties, the most common being iceberg, romaine, green and red oak, and butterhead lettuces. Due to their delicate leaves, they are prone to high pesticide use when grown conventionally, so be sure to wash them thoroughly, or better still buy organically or grow your own. Romaine lettuce is one of the most nutritious lettuce varieties and is an excellent source of vitamins A, C, K, and folate, and a very good source of manganese, potassium, molybdenum, and iron. Molybdenum's role is not well known; however, its concentrations in tooth enamel and in the liver and kidneys suggests its important role in these locations.

Pea shoots

Pea greens are clipped from the tender shoots of young pea plants, and they are delicious! The shoots are a source of vitamins A, C, E, and K, as well as B vitamins, particularly folate. Pea greens are especially rich in carotenoid antioxidants, which are important for our eye health, fertility, and the immune system. In addition, the antioxidant flavonoids quercetin and caffeic acid are present, which have anti-inflammatory and anticancer properties, respectively.

Turnip greens

Turnip greens are part of the brassica family and are significantly more nutritious than the more readily used root vegetable associated with them. Turnip greens are easy to grow from autumn through spring if the winter is relatively mild in between. Rich in vitamins A, C, and K, turnip greens also contain manganese, vitamin E, and have twice the calcium of mustard greens. They also have more cancer-fighting glucosinolates than cabbage or kale. Turnip greens are on the spicy side, so are best used in combination with another milder green in smoothies.

Watercress

Watercress, with its peppery, sour, and succulent leaves, is part of the brassica family and has all the benefits of its cousins, with its anti-ancer glucosinolates, gluconasturtiin in particular, being responsible for its peppery flavor. Watercress has an outstanding amount of vitamins C and K, and is also a great source of A, B, and E vitamins and calcium. Similar to turnip greens, the flavor of watercress is strong in a smoothie and not for the fainthearted!

THE SPRING GARDEN

In regions that have all of the traditional four seasons, the first official month of spring is the most popular time to get the year's garden planted. When starting from scratch (or if you have let your autumn and winter garden grow wild) it can be a lot of work, but rest assured it's completely worth it for those summer and autumn harvests.

Unfortunately, what you plant in spring doesn't actually give you much of anything to eat during the season. Your early spring harvest is going to consist of what you planted in winter: Asian greens, cabbage, cilantro, spinach, and turnip greens. Additionally, you will be able to harvest quick-growing greens planted in spring, such as endive, lettuce varieties, pea greens, and radish tops.

Herbs such as mint that can die off over cold winters will spring back to life, and if you have planted parsley once before, it will have gone to seed and will grow again all by itself with gusto! If you don't have your own lemon or lime tree, I recommend getting to know people who do. This is because in spring, there will be a glut of these gorgeous fruits to add zing to your green smoothies from their flesh and zest.

A Star Is Born

This Asian-inspired smoothie includes the "star" of the show: star fruit. Otherwise known as carambola, star fruit is rich in potassium and vitamin C; it packs a punch in nutrition alongside the electrolyte-rich coconut water and antioxidant-rich cilantro in this drink. Reserve a slice of star fruit for garnish—just for fun!

1 cup diced **STAR FRUITS**

½ cup **YOUNG COCONUT FLESH**

1½ cups **COCONUT WATER**

½ head **BUTTER LETTUCE**

small handful of **CILANTRO LEAVES**

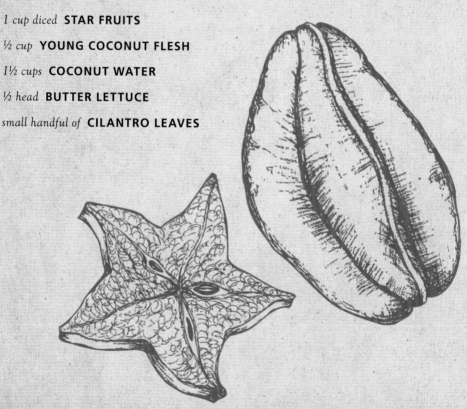

Luscious Lassi

Reminiscent of an Indian mango lassi, this smoothie is simple and stunning. Sweet and creamy, with a spicy little kick—it's almost too delicious!

2 **MANGOES**

1½ cups **ALMOND MILK**

¼ to ½ teaspoon **GROUND CARDAMOM**

squeeze of **LEMON JUICE**

big handful of **SPINACH**

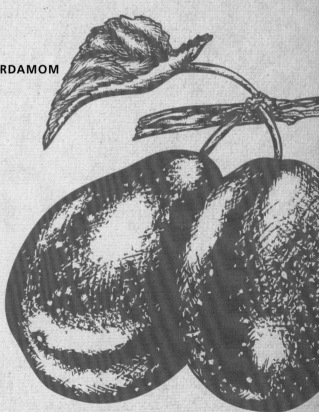

Lychee Love

Lychees have been treasured in China for over 2000 years and ought to be eaten fresh to maximize their exotic fragrance. In this smoothie, the lychee, rich in vitamin C, is complemented by the anthocyanin antioxidants in the blueberries and betalain antioxidants in the chard. If you don't have the patience to peel and seed a whole cup of lychees, try ½ cup and use extra blueberries.

1 cup peeled, seeded **LYCHEES**

1 cup **BLUEBERRIES**

1 **BANANA**

1 cup **ALMOND MILK**

2 to 3 large **SWISS OR RAINBOW CHARD**

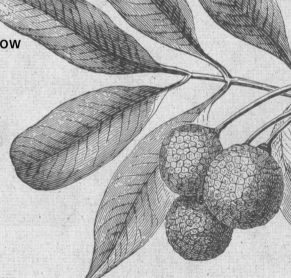

Strawberry Fields

Eating the very first strawberry of the season comes with much excitement! This luscious fruit, famous worldwide, is unfortunately one of the most heavily sprayed with pesticides, so try and buy them organic, or better still, grow your own.

2 frozen **BANANAS**, *sliced*

1 cup unhulled **STRAWBERRIES**

zest and flesh of ½ **LEMON**

1 cup **WATER OR ALMOND MILK**

AGAVE SYRUP OR HONEY, *to taste*

handful of **MINT LEAVES**

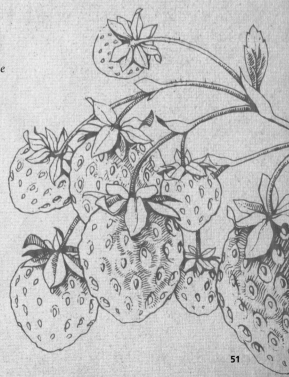

Rock Me, Baby

The marriage of melons and berries is a delight! And the simple pairing of cantaloupe (called rockmelon in some regions) and humble strawberry provides a delightful smoothie rich in vitamins A and C and the mineral manganese.

1½ cups diced **CANTALOUPE**

1 cup unhulled **STRAWBERRIES**

1 cup **WATER**

3 to 4 leaves **NAPA CABBAGE**

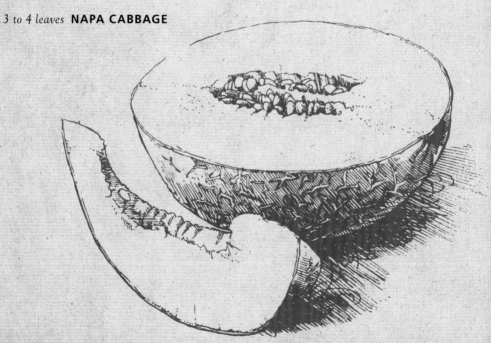

Stomach Soother

Revered as a sacred food by the ancient Egyptians, honeydew melon simply "pops" with the added zing from the ginger and lemon. A good source of vitamin B6, folate, and potassium, this smoothie could be used to relieve nausea associated with pregnancy.

2½ cups diced **HONEYDEW MELON**

1 to 2 (⅛-inch) slices **FRESH GINGER**

zest of ½ **LEMON**

1 cup **WATER**

1 to 2 handfuls of **RADISH TOPS**

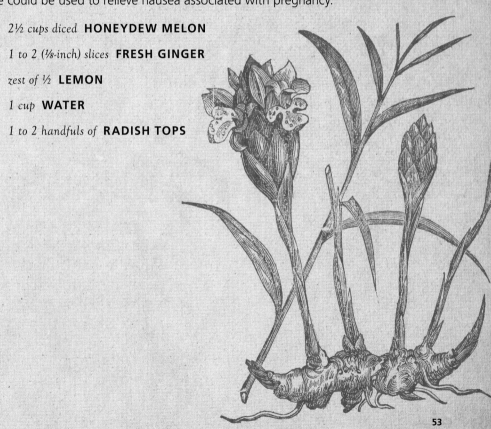

Piña Colada

Fancy a trip to Puerto Rico? No need, as this delectable smoothie is as good as the famous South American cocktail—minus the rum of course!—plus the addition of tender springtime mesclun salad mix.

1½ *cups diced* **PINEAPPLE**

flesh and water of 1 **COCONUT**

flesh of ½ **LIME**

2 *handfuls of* **MESCLUN MIX**

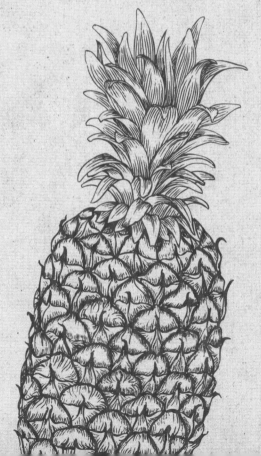

Citrus Blast

Known as one of the "seven wonders of Barbados," grapefruit is either loved or despised! Like in tomatoes, the pink and red pigments contain the highly beneficial antioxidant lycopene. The sweet mandarins, sour lemons, and bitter grapefruit complement each other to balance flavor.

1 cup diced **PINK OR RED GRAPEFRUIT**, peeled

2 **MANDARIN ORANGES**, peeled and seeded

zest and flesh of ½ **LEMON**

½ **AVOCADO**, pitted and peeled

AGAVE SYRUP OR HONEY, to taste

2 handfuls of **SPINACH**

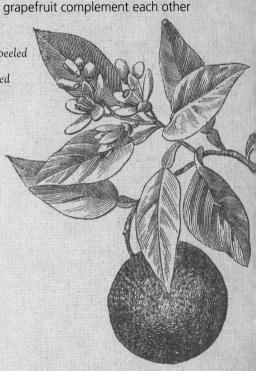

Lady Marmalade

Unlike orange-colored citrus fruits, kumquats can be eaten whole. Both kumquats and parsley are sources of iron and vitamin C, which is great because iron needs vitamin C for absorption. This is an excellent smoothie to drink during pregnancy or for anyone with anaemia.

1 cup whole **KUMQUAT** *(halved and seeded if necessary)*

1 sweet **APPLE**

1 **CUCUMBER**

1 teaspoon **VANILLA EXTRACT**

½ cup **WATER**

½ cup **ICE CUBES**

handful of **PARSLEY**

AGAVE SYRUP OR HONEY, *to taste*

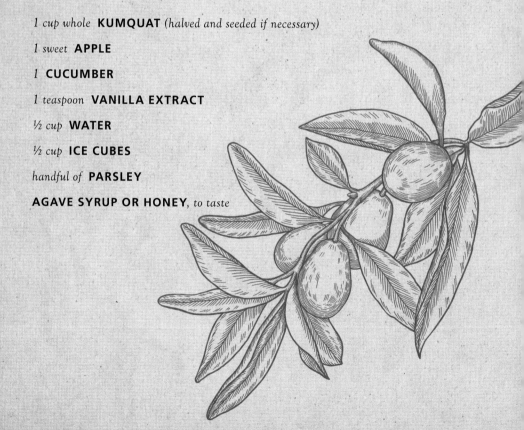

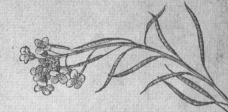

Brain Booster

Peppery and tangy, watercress is not for the fainthearted! Part of the cabbage family, watercress is antioxidant rich with high concentrations of nutrients great for immunity and eye health. It's also an outstanding source of vitamin K, which is important for our bones, blood, and brain.

2 **ORANGES**, *peeled*

1 **LIME**, *peeled*

½ **AVOCADO**, *pitted and peeled*

1½ *cups* **ORANGE JUICE**

handful of **WATERCRESS**

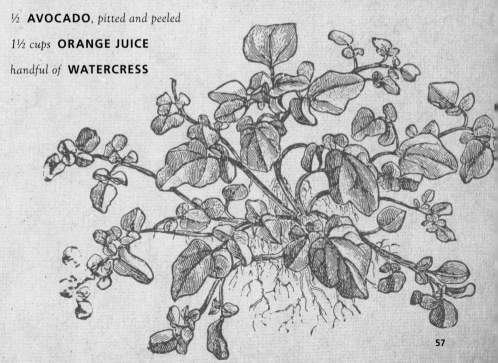

Honeymoon Healer

Cranberries may be synonymous with Christmas but they're also well known for their treatment of urinary tract infections—proanthocyanidins found in cranberries act as a barrier to bacteria in the urinary tract. How clever!

1 cup **CRANBERRIES**

1 **ORANGE**, *peeled*

zest of ½ **ORANGE**

1½ cups **ORANGE JUICE**

1 teaspoon **VANILLA EXTRACT**

pinch of **GROUND CLOVES**

6 leaves **GREEN-STEM BOK CHOY**

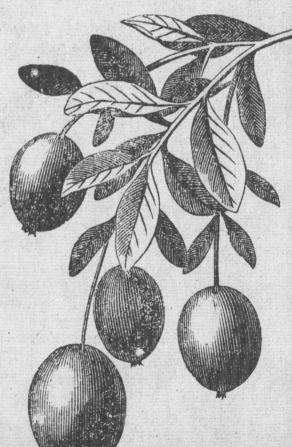

Watermelon Wow!

The delightful pairing of hydrating watermelon and antioxidant-rich raspberries is supercharged by the addition of borage, rich in anti-inflammatory omega-6 GLA, and vitamins A, C, B3, and iron.

2½ *cups* **WATERMELON**

1 *cup* **RASPBERRIES**

a squeeze of **LIME JUICE**

1 *to 2 handfuls of* **BORAGE LEAVES AND FLOWERS**

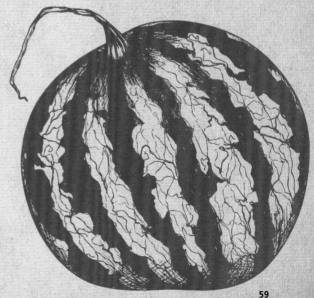

Bee Gees

This smoothie is a B-vitamin bonanza with B6 from the bananas and folate from the papaya and beet greens. Using the beet stems as well as the leaves provides colorful betalain pigments with detoxifying, antioxidant-fighting, and anti-inflammatory properties, which are maximized when eaten and blended raw.

1 cup **PAPAYA FLESH**

2 **BANANAS**

1½ cups **WATER**

6 to 8 large **BEET LEAVES AND STEMS**

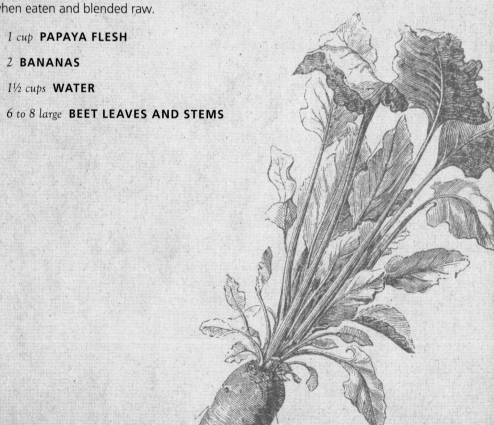

Princess and the Pea

With fewer carbs than green peas and more vitamin C and folate, sugar snaps and pea shoots are simply stunning in this savory smoothie. Rounded off with creamy avocado and finished with mint, it's the perfect springtime refresher and it's very, very green!

½ cup **SUGAR SNAP PEAS**, *stems and strings removed*

1 **AVOCADO**, *pitted and peeled*

½ cup **ICE CUBES**

1 cup **WATER**

handful of tender **PEA SHOOTS**

pinch of **SALT**

2 to 3 sprigs of **MINT**

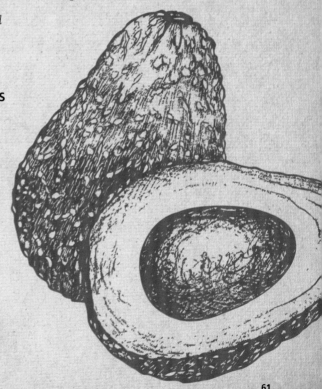

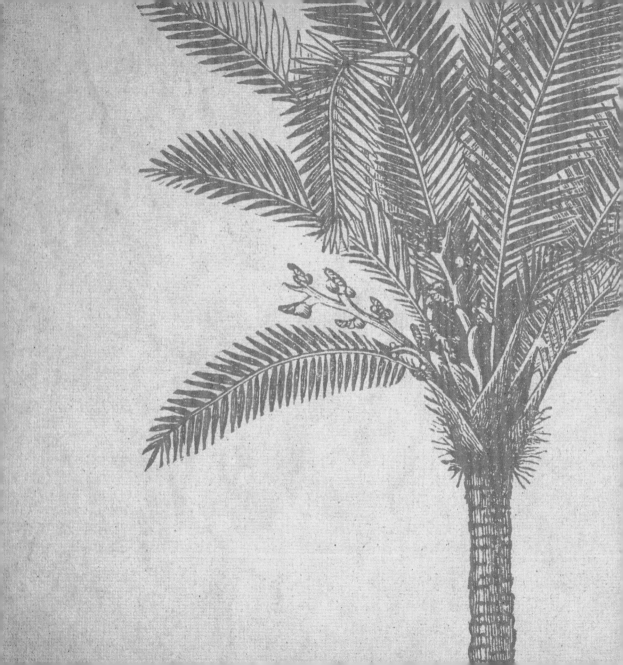

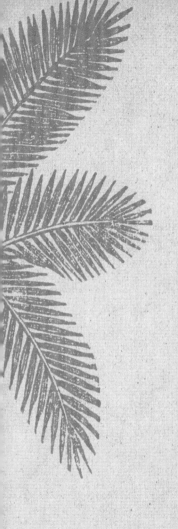

SUMMER
FUN

Summer is synonymous with luscious, sweet fruits. It is a magical time for green smoothies and also a great time to buy produce in bulk, when fruits are at their best quality and inexpensive at farmers markets. Freeze what you don't use for later in the year, when there is limited produce available and you need some extra variety.

Summer fruits provide exactly what we need for those long, hot days. Not only are peaches, melons, berries, mangoes, grapes, and cucumbers cool and refreshing, they are also water-rich and hydrating. Eat your water! The inviting summer months make us more active and we need to get extra energy from our food. The balance of fiber and natural sugars in fruit provides a sustained release of energy, and the abundance of brightly colored fruits ensures we get plenty of antioxidants to supercharge each day!

Summer is also a great time for greens, as the warmth and sun spur rapid growth. Basil, borage, celery, dandelion, lamb's-quarters, lettuce varieties, mint, parsley, purslane, strawberry leaves, and Swiss chard are classic summer greens that help to create a myriad of green smoothie combinations.

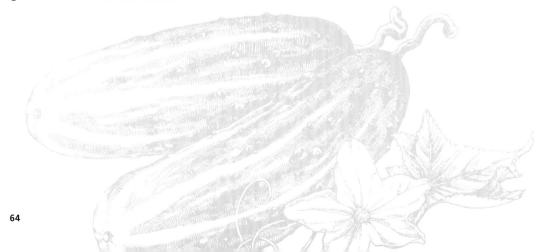

SUMMER STONE FRUIT

Otherwise known as "drupes," stone fruits all contain vitamins A, B, and C, as well as the minerals potassium, iron, magnesium, and zinc. But the benefits don't stop there—they're also rich in the phenolic antioxidants lutein and zeaxanthin, which promote eye health, particularly for the macula, which is prone to degeneration as you age.

Apricots Apricots were spread through Europe by the Greeks and have been prized since antiquity as the "golden eggs of the sun." A particularly good source of iron when dried, they are best if purchased untreated to avoid potential adverse reactions to sulphites. Untreated dried apricots will look brown, not orange.

Cherries Cherries contain deeply colored anthocyanin pigments in their skin, and their flesh contains free radical–fighting powers that are particularly good for gout and arthritis. Cherries are also rich in melatonin, a powerful antioxidant that is calming to the nervous system and helps regulate the sleep cycle.

Nectarines Nectarines are similar to a peach but without the fuzz, and the white- or orange-fleshed fruits are an excellent source of vitamin E, a fat-soluble antioxidant vitamin that is important for metabolism, the immune system, and soft-tissue healing.

Peaches Peaches were considered by the ancients to be a symbol of immortality and friendship. Like other stone fruit, peaches are a source of beta-carotene, which converts to vitamin A in the body, important for vision, mucous membranes, and glowing skin.

Plums Plums are rich in fiber, sorbitol, and isatin, which makes them a fantastic fruit for the management of constipation, particularly when dried as prunes.

BERRIES

Berries are not just delicious, they're incredibly nutritious thanks to the antioxidant power from vitamin C, phenolic flavonoids, and anthocyanin and carotenoid pigments. The phenolic "ellagic acid" in all four berries listed here is known to promote wound healing and has anticancer properties. Moreover, they contain vitamins A, B, C, and E, and trace minerals such as potassium, and particularly manganese, which assists with absorption of vitamin C.

Blackberries Blackberries contain magnesium, important for blood sugar regulation and a healthy nervous system, along with copper, which is required for bone health and the production of white and red blood cells. Particularly rich in the dark anthocyanin pigments, these berries also have anti-inflammatory and anticancer properties.

Blueberries Blueberries pack the highest amount of antioxidants of any fresh berry, according to their ORAC (oxygen radical absorbance capacity) score—particularly for eye and brain health. Also boasting antibacterial properties, blueberries have a similar effect on the urinary tract as cranberries do.

Raspberries Raspberries are similar to blackberries for their vitamin and mineral properties, and they also contain iron and magnesium. Chock-full of carotenoid pigments lutein and zeaxanthin, raspberries are also great for eye health. In addition, raspberries possess anti-aging and anti-inflammatory flavonoids such as quercetin and gallic acid.

Strawberries Strawberries are an immune-boosting powerhouse, containing more vitamin C than oranges. They're especially welcome during the muggy summer months because the vitamin B5 helps clear the skin. Strawberries are also a source of iodine, important for thyroid and potassium, and great for regulating blood pressure.

MELONS

Melons are members of the cucurbit family of plants, which also includes cucumbers, pumpkins, and squash. They are characterized by sweet, juicy flesh with high water content and a firm outer rind. Melon rinds are particularly germy (outbreaks of melon-born listeriosis have been lethal), so be sure to wash the outer rind thoroughly before cutting.

Cantaloupes
Cantaloupes, a type of muskmelon, are also known as rockmelons. They have a softer rind than other melons and light orange flesh that is very rich in beta-carotene and vitamin C. The beta-carotene content is thirty times more than in oranges. Cantaloupes are also a good source of potassium, B vitamins, and magnesium. Cantaloupes will continue to ripen once picked and should have a sweet, fragrant smell that is not overpowering.

Honeydew melons
Honeydew melon is also a variety of muskmelon. Reportedly Napoleon's favorite fruit, honeydew has a pale green, creamy rind with light green flesh. This melon is an excellent source of potassium; it is also vital for cellular health, the nervous system, and preventing and lowering high blood pressure. Buy your honeydews ripe, as these non-climacteric fruit don't continue to ripen after picking.

Watermelons
Watermelon, also a non-climacteric fruit, needs to be purchased ripe to maximize both its nutritional benefits and taste. The deep pink flesh of vitamin C–rich watermelon is due to the pigment lycopene, which is important for bone and cardiovascular health. Watermelon also contains the triterpenoid, "cucurbitacin E," a potent anti-inflammatory agent. Of further benefit to cardiovascular health is the excellent amount of the amino acid citrulline, which converts to arginine in the body.

SUMMER GREENS

Like spring, summer is an abundant time for greenery, bringing powerhouses of flavor and nutrition with edible weeds and flowers that will likely grow all by themselves in your back garden if you haven't planted them yourself.

Borage Borage is a native plant of Europe and also known as the "bee plant," given it attracts numerous bees to its beautiful purple, star-shaped flowers. Easy to grow and very nutritious, borage is chock-full of B vitamins, particularly B3, as well vitamins A and C. Borage is great for women's health as it is a good source of iron, calcium, magnesium, and zinc. Borage is also uniquely rich in GLA (gamma-linolenic-acid), which gets converted to the anti-inflammatory fatty acid DGLA in the body. The conversion requires nutrients such as magnesium, zinc, and vitamins C and B3—exactly what borage contains! Not only does the fatty acid fight inflammation, it's also good for skin, allergies, joints, and the brain, and it's great for kids due to its role with growth, development, and behavior.

Dandelions Dandelions are well known for their use as a liver tonic due to their rich antioxidant phytochemicals such as the bitter sesquiterpenes, and anti-inflammatory apigenin and luteolin. Dandelions are also rich in anti-bacterial gallic acid and gut- and blood-detoxifying fibrous pectins. They are also, surprisingly, the richest plant source of beta-carotene, and also contain vitamins B, C, E, and K, along with choline, potassium, iron, calcium, magnesium, phosphorus, copper, cobalt, zinc, boron, and molybdenum. They are a trace mineral goldmine! Of course, you'll need to use these spicy-bitter, flavor-filled leaves sparingly. Try balancing them with another milder green.

Lamb's-Quarters Also known as wild spinach, lamb's-quarters are widely considered a weed due to their often prolific growth just about anywhere. But this weed is a treasure unto itself—lamb's-quarters are a highly nutritious green related to spinach and quinoa. And like quinoa, they are a complete protein! They are rich in vitamins A, B, C, and K, along with minerals such as calcium, manganese, iron, magnesium, phosphorus, and potassium.

Purslane Purslane is also a nutritious edible weed, characterized by succulent red/green stems and green leaves. Purslane has the richest source of omega-3 ALA in a leafy green. Its red and yellow betalain pigments are also anticancer antioxidants. In addition, purslane contains vitamins A, B, C, and E along with magnesium, iron, calcium, potassium, and manganese. Both the stems and leaves can be eaten and used in green smoothies.

Strawberry leaves Eaten fresh or steeped in tea, strawberry leaves have long been used as a remedy for digestive distress such as nausea, bloating, and diarrhea. Nutritionally, strawberry leaves are known to contain iron, calcium, and vitamin C, and their antioxidant phytochemicals are stronger than those in the fruit, namely caffeic acid, which is good for reducing inflammation in swollen arthritic joints, and ellagic acid, known for its anticancer and wound-healing properties. If you can't access fresh strawberry leaves (which usually means growing them yourself), at least leave the hulls on when blending strawberries into your smoothies.

TENDING THE SUMMER GARDEN

Early summertime means berries! Strawberries, raspberries, blueberries, and blackberries are producing their first, sweet crops and offer an unrivaled base for your smoothie recipes. Green smoothie–friendly vegetables, planted in spring and late winter, are also ready for harvest. These include celery, cucumbers, and tomatoes, and the green tops from beets and radishes.

To ensure an adequate and ongoing supply of leafy greens, be sure to plant lettuce varieties every few weeks. Lettuce needs plenty of sun and water to grow quickly, which is doubly necessary since slow-growing lettuce greens will be bitter and will go to seed.

Herbs like basil, mint, and borage grow beautifully in summer and can be harvested from the same plants continuously. Easy-to-grow Swiss chard can also be harvested from the same plant over and over by cutting off outer, mature leaves.

In areas prone to high heat, try to plant your garden where there is some late afternoon shade, and avoid planting alongside brick walls that retain and radiate heat. If planting in pots like I do, you can move your plants around to avoid the extreme heat of certain days.

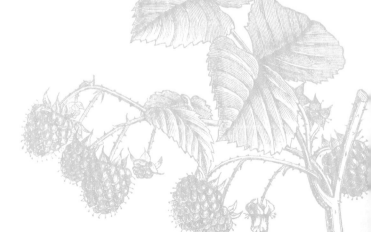

Sweet Summertime

Also known as wild spinach, fat hen, and goosefoot, lamb's-quarters are an edible weed rich in vitamins C, A, and K. They are also very high in kidney stone–causing oxalates, so use them infrequently in green smoothies. With its gorgeous summer stone fruit and spices, this smoothie has it going on!

1½ cups **APRICOT AND PEACH FLESH**

1 small frozen **BANANA**, sliced

1 teaspoon **VANILLA EXTRACT**

½ teaspoon **GROUND CINNAMON**

a pinch of **GROUND CARDAMOM**

1½ cups **ALMOND MILK**

handful of **LAMB'S-QUARTERS**

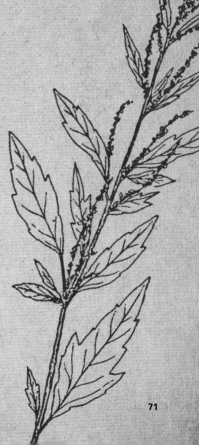

Moving and Grooving

Chia seeds are an Aztec superfood rich in omega-3 ALA, calcium, magnesium, and are a complete protein source. Use chia seeds to thicken a runny smoothie if desired, or to add extra soluble and insoluble fiber to aid bowel health and blood sugar regulation.

3½ cups diced **WATERMELON**

1 to 2 (⅛-inch) slices **FRESH GINGER**

1 to 2 tablespoons **CHIA SEEDS** (optional)

handful of **MINT**

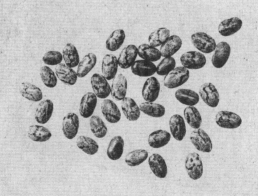

B6 Bombshell

Vitamin B6 is essential for our blood and immune and nervous systems. Thankfully, this smoothie is jam-packed with it! In addition, chard is an incredible source of vitamins A and K, and is rich in minerals, including iron, magnesium, and manganese.

1 **MANGO**

1 **BANANA**

1 **ORANGE**, *peeled*

1½ cups **WATER OR ALMOND MILK**

handful of **SWISS OR RAINBOW CHARD**

Strawberry Sensation

This decadent smoothie is like a thick strawberry shake—perfect for a summer morning before the heat of the day strikes or as a delightful dessert.

1 cup unhulled **FRESH STRAWBERRIES**

1 cup **FROZEN STRAWBERRIES**

½ cup **RAW CASHEWS**

1 cup **COCONUT WATER**

small handful of **STRAWBERRY LEAVES**

a few **BASIL LEAVES**

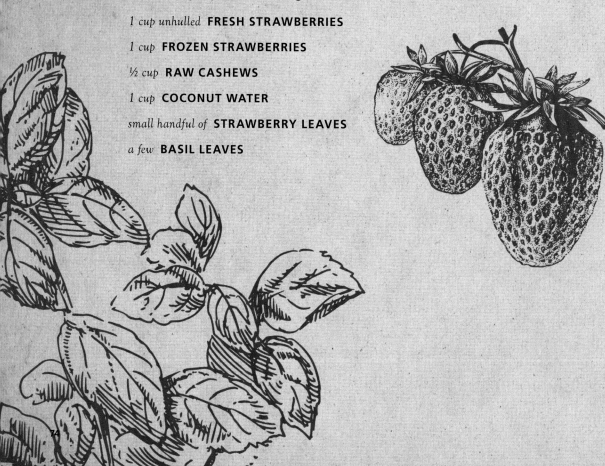

Enzyme Frenzy

Anti-inflammatory is the word! With celery's non-starch polysaccharides, bromelain from the pineapple, and protein-digesting enzymes from the papaya, this smoothie is perfect for anyone with arthritis.

¾ cup **PAPAYA FLESH**

¾ cup diced **PINEAPPLE**

handful of pale **CELERY LEAVES**

a few **PINEAPPLE SAGE LEAVES** (optional)

1½ cups **WATER**

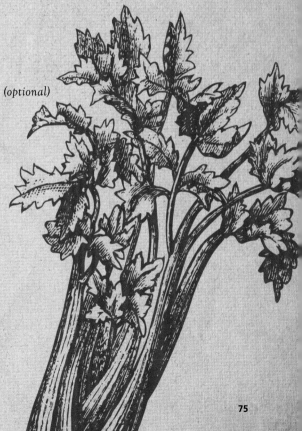

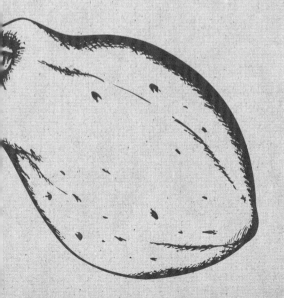

Groovy Grapes

A summer delight. Sweet, fresh, antioxidant- and vitamin-rich grapes and melons balance the powerful flavor of iron-packed parsley.

1½ cups **RED OR GREEN SEEDLESS GRAPES**

2 cups diced **MELON** (any variety)

6 to 8 **GREEN OAK LETTUCE LEAVES**

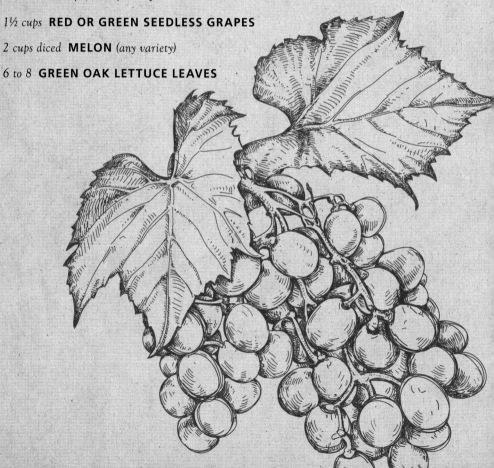

A Taste of Mexico

Guava, agave, coconut, and lime will get your taste buds tingling in this Mexican-inspired drink! Succulent fresh purslane often grows wild and abundantly in many home gardens. It's worth identifying for use as it has the highest omega-3 ALA content of any leafy plant. In late summer, look for feijoa (pineapple guava).

1 cup **GUAVA**

flesh and water of 1 **YOUNG COCONUT**

zest and juice of 1 **LEMON OR LIME**

1 to 2 handfuls of **PURSLANE**

AGAVE SYRUP, to taste

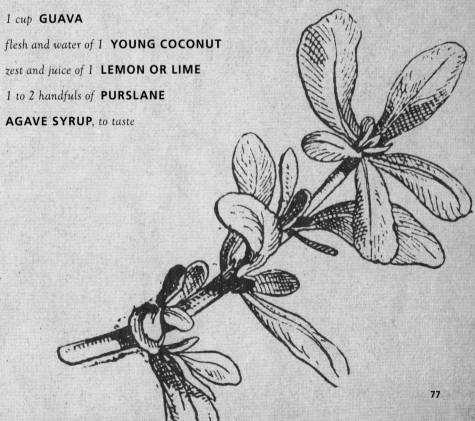

Chillax with Cherries

In addition to being rich in pain-relieving anthocyanins, cherries contain high levels of melatonin, a hormone that helps us to relax and sleep. Partnered with GLA-rich borage flowers, also known as starflower, it creates an antioxidant and anti-inflammatory powerhouse of a green smoothie!

1 cup pitted **CHERRIES**

1 frozen **BANANA**, *sliced*

½ teaspoon **GROUND CINNAMON**

1½ cups **COCONUT WATER**

1 to 2 handfuls of **BORAGE LEAVES AND FLOWERS**

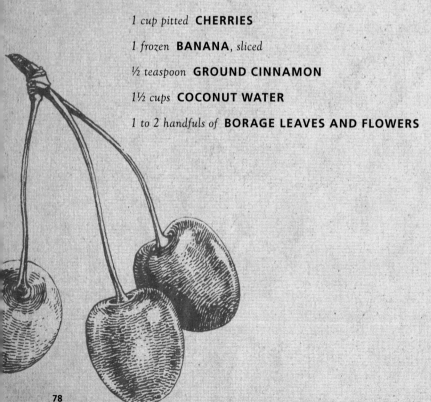

Berry Blast

Blueberries and raspberries are both delicious, antioxidant-rich fruits best enjoyed at the height of summer. Even richer in vitamins is the gorgeous, crisp romaine lettuce that gives the smoothie its "green."

2 frozen **BANANAS**, *sliced*

1 cup **RASPBERRIES OR BLUEBERRIES**

1½ cups **WATER OR ALMOND MILK**

1 to 2 handfuls of **ROMAINE LETTUCE**

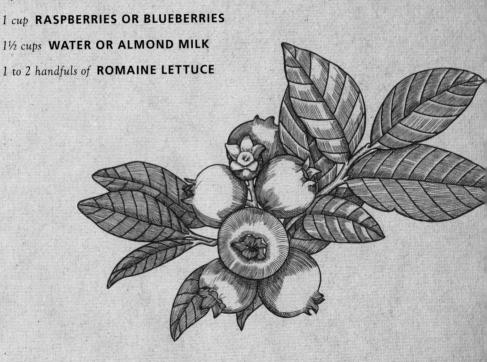

4Ps

Papaya—rich in protein-digesting enzymes.

Pineapple—an excellent source of manganese, essential to activate many enzyme reactions.

Passionfruit—a great source of dietary fiber and simply delicious to garnish a smoothie.

Parsley—the great detoxifier with very high antioxidant flavonoids and pigments like chlorophyll.

1 cup **PAPAYA FLESH**

1 cup diced **PINEAPPLE**

handful of **PARSLEY**

1½ cups **WATER**

flesh of 2 **PASSIONFRUITS** (stir through finished smoothie by hand)

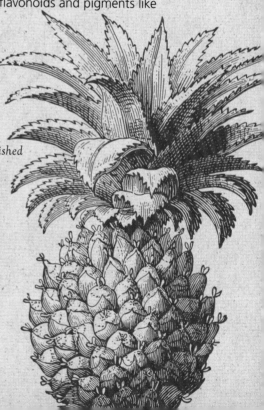

Just Peachy

Nothing says summer like mangoes and peaches! With the ice cream–like feature of frozen banana and the subtle flavor of butter lettuce, this is a great introduction to green smoothies.

flesh of 1 **MANGO**

1 **PEACH**

1 frozen **BANANA**, *sliced*

1 cup **WATER OR ALMOND MILK**

1 head **BUTTER LETTUCE**

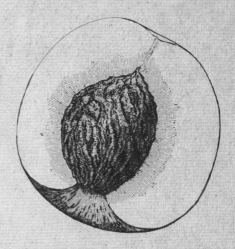

Pacific Sunset

This smooth, silky, and creamy smoothie offers the perfect way to end summer with two of the season's most prized stone fruits. Dandelion greens, cheap and nutrient-packed summer leaves, lend a spicy twist to wake up the whole body.

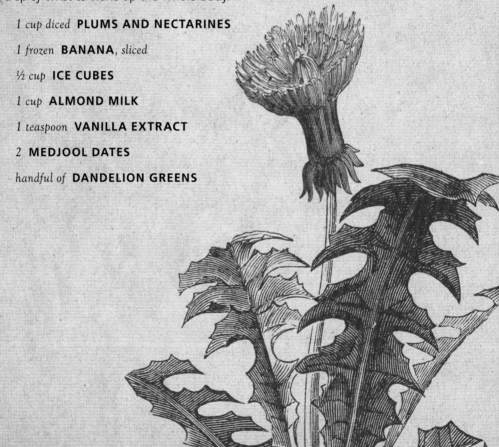

1 cup diced **PLUMS AND NECTARINES**

1 frozen **BANANA**, *sliced*

½ cup **ICE CUBES**

1 cup **ALMOND MILK**

1 teaspoon **VANILLA EXTRACT**

2 **MEDJOOL DATES**

handful of **DANDELION GREENS**

Insalata Caprese Green Smoothie

Paying homage to the days before I developed a dairy intolerance, *insalata caprese*, a dish of mozzarella, tomatoes, and basil, is a salad I used to enjoy. Let's just switch the cheese for papaya and we have a hit! It's a little bit sweet and a little bit savory; you choose at which time of the day this smoothie suits you.

1 cup **PAPAYA FLESH**

1½ cups diced **TOMATOES**

1 cup **WATER**

small handful of **BASIL**

dash of **EXTRA-VIRGIN OLIVE OIL**

pinch of **SALT**

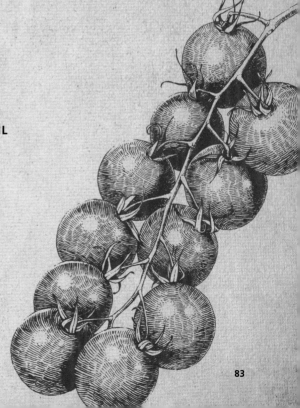

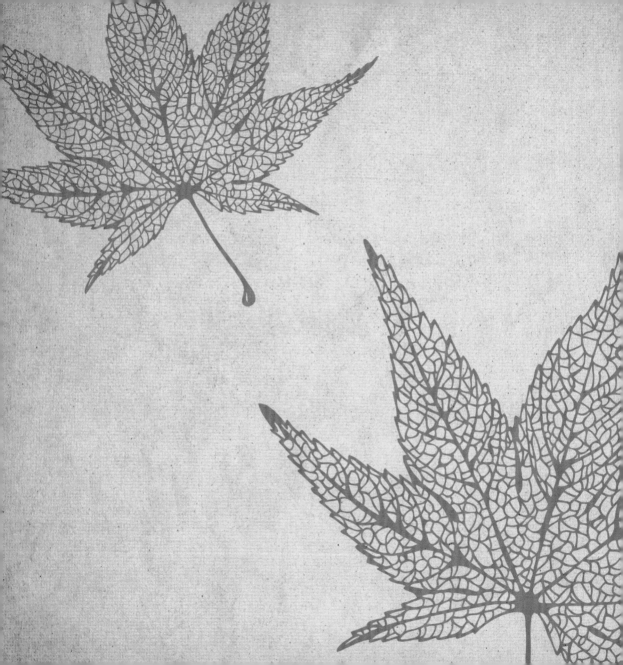

FALL INTO AUTUMN

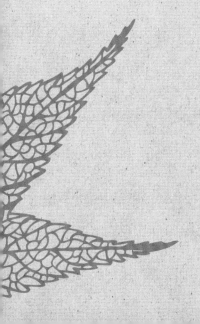

Like spring, autumn is such a beautiful and colorful time of the year, as the hot summer transitions to mild sunny days and cool nights, and the deciduous foliage undergoes spectacular color changes. One of the other reasons autumn is my favorite time of the year is the sensational variety of produce available.

Early autumn has the tail end of beautiful summer fruits like strawberries, nectarines, plums, peaches, grapes, and melons, while new-season fruits like apples, pears, kiwi, and citrus make a long-awaited return. Guava, figs, and passionfruit make appearances in autumn, as do persimmons and pomegranates as winter approaches. The huge variety of fruits available in autumn helps with the creation of an amazing variety of delicious combinations of green smoothies.

Nutritious autumn greens include Asian greens, basil, beet greens, collards, celery, cilantro, endive, fennel tops, kale, lettuce varieties, mint, parsley, radish tops, and Swiss chard.

AUTUMN FRUITS

Green smoothies are never dull in autumn, with variety like no other time of the year.

Apples   The soluble fiber pectin, rich in apples, is important for lowering cholesterol and encourages growth of good bacteria in the bowel. As well as B and C vitamins, apples contain the mineral boron, important for bone health. Apples also contain antioxidants such as anti-inflammatory quercetin, insulin-mimicking epicatechin, and procyanidin B2, which is good for scalp health.

Pears   Considered one of the least allergenic fruits available, pears are used for elimination-type diets (with the exception of those with fructose malabsorption; pears as well as apples are not suitable for this type of digestive disorder). Rich in soluble and insoluble fiber, pears are fantastic for bowel health to keep things moving, and the gritty fiber helps to remove toxins from the gut.

Figs   Native to Turkey, figs are a source of vitamins A, E, K, and B-group vitamins. They also contain potent flavonoid antioxidants such as chlorogenic acid, which is useful in blood sugar regulation. Minerals such as calcium, iron, selenium, and zinc are known to be more concentrated in dried figs. Only available fresh for a short time, this delicate fruit is not to be missed.

Kiwi   Famously grown in New Zealand, and also known as the Chinese gooseberry, kiwi are China's national fruit. Abundantly rich in vitamin C, kiwis are a great source of soluble fiber, and the seeds are rich in omega-3 alpha-linolenic acid (ALA). Kiwis are also a source of vitamins A, C, and E, antioxidant flavonoids, potassium, magnesium, manganese, and iron.

Passionfruits Originating in South America and otherwise known as the granadilla, passionfruits contain edible seeds that are covered in juicy, membranous sacs. Containing antioxidants beta-carotene and cryptoxanthin-B, passionfruits are nutritionally good for eye health. These delicious fruits also contain B and C vitamins, iron, copper, manganese, and phosphorus. They are available all year round, but are most abundant in late summer and autumn.

Guavas/feijoas Guava has pink flesh colored by lycopene, and the feijoa (otherwise known as a pineapple guava) has yellow flesh. Both are rich in soluble fiber, vitamin C, and antioxidants such as macular protective carotenoids. Pink guava contains twice the lycopene as tomatoes, which protects the skin from UV damage and is good for the prostate. It also contains B vitamins, vitamins E and K, magnesium, and manganese.

Grapes Botanically known as berries, huge varieties are grown for eating or wine making. The red or purple grape pigments from anthocyanins, and the green from catechins, are both anti-inflammatory and antiallergenic in nature. Grapes are also known for their resveratrol content, which protects against colon and prostate cancers, heart disease, and neurological disorders.

Persimmons Rich in antimicrobial and anti-inflammatory catechins and gallocatechins, persimmons are delicious, vitamin- and mineral-rich fruits available in many varieties, some of which originate from China and some from North America. Persimmons contain betulinic acid, which has antitumor properties, lycopene pigments to give it its orange color, and are also rich in zeaxanthin for macular (eye) health.

AUTUMN GREENS

Early autumn greens reflect the end of summer, with fragrant herbs, edible weeds, and lettuce varieties still available. Subsequently, the availability of fall greenery transitions into cooler climate leaves such as the Asian greens and kale, which are chock-full of antioxidants to bolster our immune systems in preparation for winter.

Asian greens There are many Asian greens, but the most common and green smoothie–friendly is bok choy, otherwise known as Chinese cabbage or pak choy. With succulent leaf bases, the green-stem variety of bok choy is mild in flavor and has more carotenoid antioxidants than other members of the brassica family. Bok choy, like other brassicas, contains anticancer and anti-inflammatory glucosinolates, as well as vitamins C, K, and B-group vitamins.

Beet greens Beet roots, stems, and leaves are all nutritional powerhouses, containing B vitamins, especially folate, as well as iron, magnesium, manganese, and potassium. Beets' folate content in combination with their betaine means beets are great for reducing homocysteine and hence are fantastic for cardiovascular, neurological, and hormone health. The red pigments in beets come from betalains, which are important antioxidant phytochemicals that facilitate glutathione function for phase II detox in the liver. Betalains are affected by heat, so for maximal benefit they should be eaten or blended raw. The leaves of beets have significantly more vitamin C and lutein carotenoids than the root, making them powerfully anti-inflammatory.

Endive   Also known as escarole, endive looks like a curly leaf green lettuce; it is different from Belgian endive, also known as witlof. Available all year round, the somewhat bitter endive is related to the daisy family. Rich in beta-carotene, vitamins C and K, B vitamins, manganese, iron, and potassium, endive is known to be good for clear skin, and its high inulin and fiber content means it is good for blood sugar regulation, lowering cholesterol, and is a good remedy for constipation.

Radish tops   As a member of the brassica family, radishes contain cancer-fighting glucosinolates and sulphur-based compounds great for liver and digestive health. Radish leaves are surprisingly mild in flavor and, given their slightly prickly surface, blend well into a smoothie. The leaves are also a richer source of iron, calcium, vitamin C, and phosphorous than the hotter-in-flavor root, as well as a source of magnesium, folate, and vitamins A, C, and K.

Chard   Related to spinach and quinoa, chard may be found with white stems (Swiss chard) or with colored stems (rainbow chard). Similar to beet greens nutritionally, chard contains betalain pigments, best eaten raw for their liver detox benefits. The presence of vitamin K, calcium, and magnesium make chard great for bone health. In addition, it contains excellent amounts of vitamins A, C, E, manganese, potassium, and iron. Chard also contains at least 13 polyphenol antioxidants, such as syringic acid, which is good for blood sugar regulation.

THE AUTUMN GARDEN

A time for the most abundant harvests, autumn is the classic time of the year for traditional harvest festivals and celebrations. Late-summer fruits and new-season autumn fruits can be bought economically in bulk, and can be preserved for later months by drying or freezing (see page 108).

For some, the home garden is harvested and cleared until it is replanted in spring. However, autumn is the perfect time to plant for winter in regions with milder climates, especially in April for the Southern Hemisphere and October in the Northern Hemisphere. Asian greens, cabbages, cilantro, kale, celery, fennel, turnips, and spinach can be planted for their smoothie-friendly greenery made available in the colder months.

Peach Melba

The peach Melba is a classic dessert created in the late 19th century by renowned French chef Escoffier to honor the Australian opera singer Dame Nellie Melba. This version omits the ice cream and of course has added greenery. It's an absolute delight!

1 cup **PEACH FLESH**

1 to 2 teaspoons **VANILLA EXTRACT**

1 cup **WATER**

½ cup **RAW CASHEWS**

6 to 8 **GREEN LETTUCE LEAVES**

1 cup **RASPBERRIES** *and 1 tablespoon* **AGAVE SYRUP OR HONEY** (*crush together by hand and stir through finished smoothie for a swirled effect*)

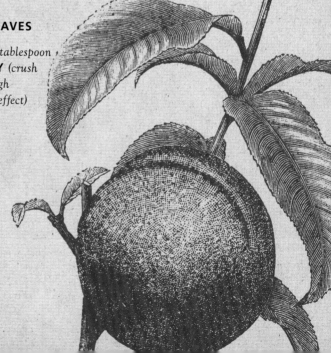

Fig-tastic

A fantastic source of minerals like iron and calcium, fresh figs have a short season, so be sure not to miss out on this amazing fruit. Classically teamed with grapes, cinnamon, and walnuts, this smoothie is an autumnal taste sensation.

5 fresh **FIGS** (or 5 dried figs, soaked in water overnight)

1½ cups **RED GRAPES**

½ teaspoon **GROUND CINNAMON**

1 cup **WATER**

6 **WALNUT HALVES**

2 to 3 **COLLARD LEAVES**

Mint and Melon Multivitamin

This simple and totally refreshing green smoothie is highlighted by mint, rich in menthols to soothe the intestines and rosmarinic acid to soothe inflamed airways, and is a source of omega-3s, vitamins A, C, E, and K, folate and vitamin B2, and iron, potassium, magnesium, manganese, *and* calcium. Simply amazing!

3 cups diced **HONEYDEW MELON**

1 cup **ICE CUBES**

1 to 2 handfuls of **MINT**

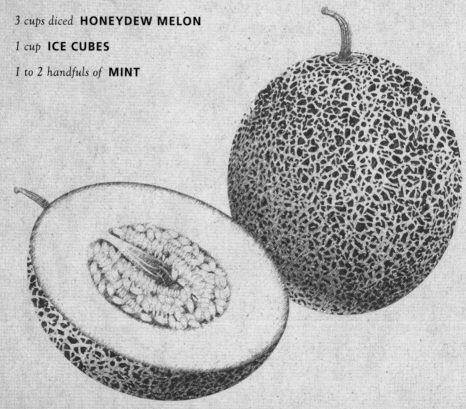

Fuyu Fever

Fuyu persimmons can be eaten firm or soft; however, for smoothies, they're a lot better when ripe and soft. This non-astringent variety of persimmon partners well with fats, such as the almond and avocado used in this recipe.

1 cup ripe (non-astringent) **FUYU PERSIMMON FLESH**

½ **AVOCADO**

1 cup **ALMOND MILK**

1 cup **WATER**

AGAVE SYRUP OR HONEY, *to taste*

3 to 4 **NAPA CABBAGE LEAVES**

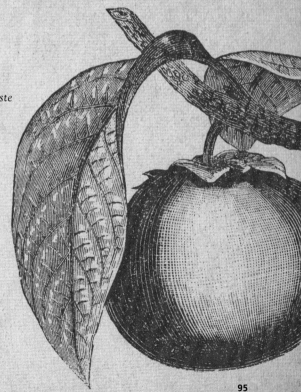

Hachiya Heaven

Hachiya is an astringent variety of persimmon that *must* be totally gooey to eat without feeling like you have a mouthful of cotton wool! Hachiya persimmon pairs well with acidic fruit, and this smoothie is packed with vitamin C and carotenoids that benefit eye health.

1 cup very, very ripe **HACHIYA PERSIMMON FLESH**

zest of ½ **LEMON**

1 **LEMON**, *peeled*

1 **LIME**, *peeled*

½ cup **ICE CUBES**

1 cup **WATER**

1 head **BUTTER LETTUCE**

AGAVE SYRUP OR HONEY, *to taste*

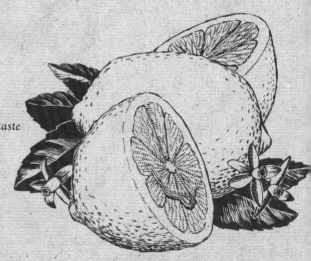

Pear Passion

Like a cross between an apple and a pear, Asian pears (or Nashi pears), are ripened on the tree and are firm when eaten. Asian pears are a delightful addition to salads and also make a very refreshing green smoothie.

2 **ASIAN PEARS**

1 **BANANA**

1½ cups **WATER OR ALMOND MILK**

2 to 3 leaves **SWISS OR RAINBOW CHARD**

flesh of 2 **PASSIONFRUITS** (*stir through finished smoothie by hand*)

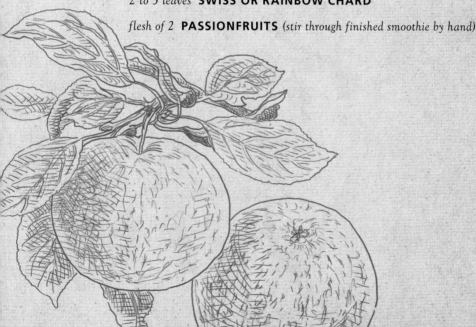

Don't Worry, Be Happy!

Nutrition plays and integral role in our brain function and mood, and this mood-enhancing green smoothie full of autumn goodies is chock-full of what we need to feel great, including vitamin B6, healthy fats, choline, folate, zinc, antioxidants, magnesium, protein, and chromium. Adding the AFA algae is optional, but it does contain PEA (phenylethylamine), the "love chemical," to give you that extra bit of bliss!

2 **BANANAS**

¼ **AVOCADO**

¼ cup mixed **SUNFLOWER AND HEMP SEEDS**

4 **MEDJOOL DATES**

2 tablespoons raw **CACAO POWDER**

1½ cups **WATER**

handful of **MINT**

1 tablespoon **AFA ALGAE** (optional)

Detox Diva

As summer's harvest spills into autumn, the last of the stone fruit can still be savored. While most sweet fruits have vitamins A and C, nectarines also contain vitamins E and B. Endive, a bitter green, is a great source of folate and choline, so all in all, this is a delightful liver-detoxifying smoothie!

1 cup **NECTARINE FLESH**

1 **BANANA**

flesh and zest of ½ **LEMON**

2 (⅛-inch) slices fresh **GINGER**

1½ cups **WATER**

handful of **ENDIVE LEAVES**

4 **MEDJOOL DATES**

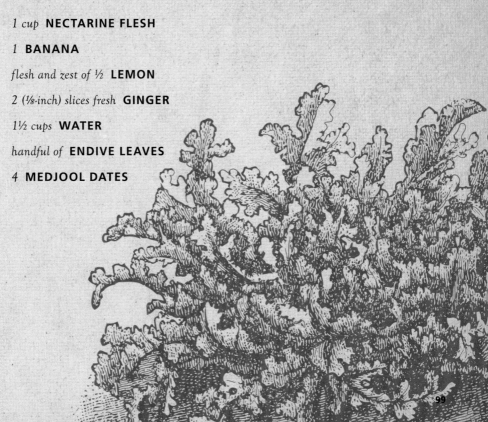

Superman

Wonderful radishes are available all year around. The leaves are quite mild, and have six times the vitamin C of the spicy-flavored root, *and* they're a source of calcium. Also including peaches, a rich iron source, this smoothie is bursting with vitamin and mineral goodness!

1 frozen **BANANA**, *sliced*

1 cup **PEACH FLESH**

½ to 1 teaspoon **GROUND CINNAMON**

1½ cups **WATER**

1 handful of **RADISH TOPS**

Pomegranate Pop

As each delightful pomegranate seed pops between your teeth, the explosion of flavor and goodness is astounding. But those seeds contain a lot more than flavor—they're chock-full of antioxidants, vitamins C and K, B-group vitamins, and many minerals. This smoothie is a taste and texture sensation!

3 **ORANGES**, *peeled*

handful of **PARSLEY**

1 cup **WATER**

4 **WALNUT HALVES**

4 **MEDJOOL DATES**

seeds from 1 large **POMEGRANATE**
(stir through finished smoothie by hand)

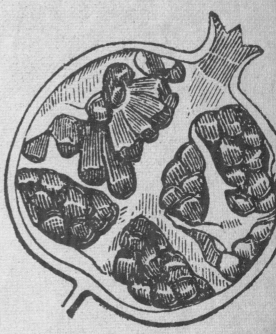

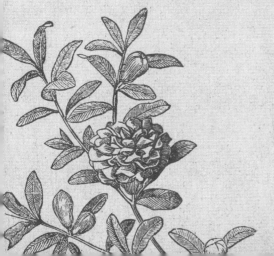

Plum Bonanza

As part of the brassica family, kale's superfood features include its glucosinolates, which help detoxify the body and lower risk of bladder, colon, ovarian, breast, and prostate cancers. With luscious, vitamin-rich plums, this smoothie is a sure-fire immune booster.

1½ cups **PLUM FLESH**

zest of ¼ **ORANGE**

3 to 4 tablespoons **HEMP SEEDS**

1 teaspoon **VANILLA EXTRACT**

1 cup **ALMOND MILK**

½ cup **ICE CUBES**

AGAVE SYRUP OR HONEY, to taste

1 to 2 handfuls of **KALE**

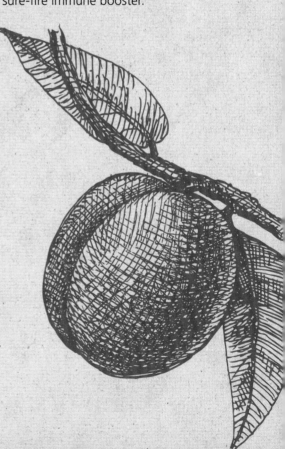

Skin Savior

This refreshing smoothie is packed with beautifying ingredients. Including silicon from the , vitamin E from the avocado, vitamin A from the figs, anti-inflammatory aloe vera, hydrating coconut water, and alkaline greens, this drink will help you get the glow.

4 to 5 fresh **FIGS** (or 4 to 5 dried figs, soaked in water overnight)

1 **CUCUMBER**

inner leaf gel of 4 inches **ALOE VERA**

1 cup **COCONUT WATER**

½ **AVOCADO**

handful of inner **CELERY LEAVES**

2 to 3 **SPRIGS MINT**

Mellow Yellow

Chock-full of bioflavonoids and carotenoids, all things yellow will supercharge your skin and eye health as well as boost your immune system in preparation for winter. This savory smoothie will tantalize the taste buds and has a beautiful golden glow!

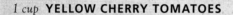

1 cup **YELLOW CHERRY TOMATOES**

1 **YELLOW BELL PEPPER**, *seeded*

½ **AVOCADO**

scant ¼ teaspoon **GROUND TURMERIC**

pinch of **CAYENNE PEPPER**

squeeze of **LEMON JUICE**

1 cup **WATER**

½ cup **ICE CUBES**

pinch of **SALT**

6 leaves **GREEN-STEM BOK CHOY**

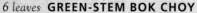

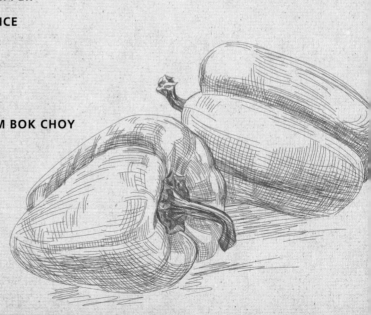

THE WINTER WONDERLAND

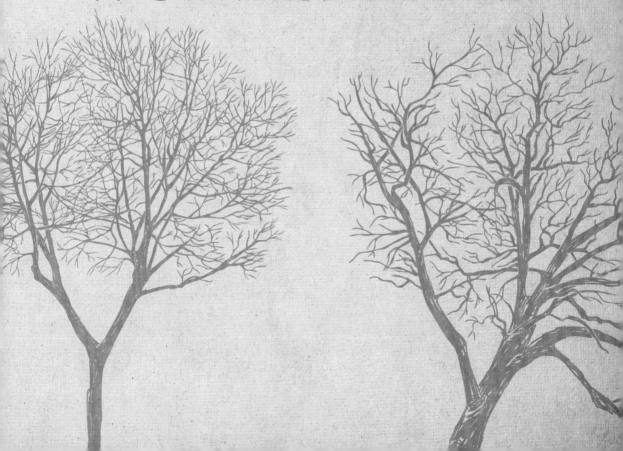

Compared with the abundance of summer and autumn fruits, winter produce can certainly present a challenge when it comes to green smoothies. However, it also can be a time for creativity. Spices such as ginger, cinnamon, and cardamom are fantastic additions to help warm you up on a cold and frosty morning.

Fats in the form of nuts, seeds, and avocado can add a more filling element to a winter green smoothie to provide plenty of sustenance throughout the day. The use of ice and frozen fruit is best avoided in smoothies at this time of year, given the weather is cold enough as it is! If frozen ingredients are used or required, be sure to blend thoroughly or thaw prior to using to avoid the potential digestive distress of a cold smoothie in cold weather.

In winter there is an abundance of citrus available, which can't be a coincidence given our need for nutrients like vitamin C and to help ward off coughs and colds. In addition to being the season that produces classic winter staples—which are rich in fiber, have a hearty texture, and make for filling, satisfying smoothies—winter is also a time for special fruits like persimmons, tamarillos, and pomegranates, which contain high levels of vitamins and antioxidants and are brilliant for unique smoothie recipes.

Nutritious winter greens can include Asian greens, beet greens, cabbage, celery, cilantro, fennel tops, kale, parsley, radish tops, spinach, Swiss chard, and turnip greens.

WINTER FRUITS

Give colds and the flu the boot with vitamin-rich winter fruits!

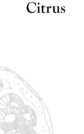

Citrus   Grapefruit, lemons, limes, mandarins, oranges, and tangelos all contain antioxidant liminoids, which are potent anticarcinogens. They possess potassium, B vitamins, cardiovascular-friendly hesperidin and hydroxycinnamic acids, and calcium and phosphorus for bone health. The majority of vitamin C is in citrus juice; the white pith contains bioflavonoids that enhance the effect of vitamin C, while seeds have anti-fungal and antibacterial qualities, and the peels of lemons and limes not only taste amazing, but are beneficial to reduce bad estrogens in our body that come from plastics and pollution.

Pomegranates   Historically a symbol of fertility, pomegranates are a unique fruit comprising multiple little seeds surrounded by a jewel of red, juicy flesh. Pomegranates are bursting with antioxidants, such as anthocyanin pigments with their anticancer properties and a polyphenol called punicalagin, which plays an important role in cardiovascular health. Pomegranates are also prized for their role in men's health, being great for the prostate, and in women's health because their phytoestrogens assist with menopausal symptoms.

Tamarillos   Also known as tree tomatoes, tamarillos are members of the nightshade family along with tomatoes, peppers, and potatoes. Rich in vitamin C and the flavonoid pigments anthocyanins and lycopene, tamarillos have significant immune-boosting antioxidant power. Tamarillos also have vitamins A, B1, B6, and E, potassium, manganese, copper, selenium, phosphorus, boron, zinc, iron, chromium, and molybdenum.

PRESERVING FRUITS FOR WINTER

Seasonal winter fruit is limited when compared to the bountiful options at other times of the year. Consider preserving fruits from late summer and autumn to add more variety to your winter smoothies. Options for preserving fruits raw are freezing and drying.

A food dehydrator (such as the nine-tray Excalibur, the best quality dehydrator on the market), can dry fruits at low temperatures, retaining their nutritional status as raw foods by heating no higher than 118°F (48°C). Any fruit can be dehydrated, and times vary according to the size of the whole or sliced fruit. Dried fruits can then be stored in the pantry for snacks, or rehydrated overnight in water to add to smoothies the next day.

Fruits such as berries, peaches, and mangoes freeze really well, as it doesn't matter that they are soft when thawed to blend into smoothies. This is good in winter when you don't want to add too many frozen ingredients to your smoothie. Peeled bananas freeze well, but when thawed they are floppy and ooze liquid, which isn't pleasant. Bananas will blend best when they're still frozen to provide an ice cream–like flavor. For apples and pears, I blend them into a puree with some lemon juice (to reduce browning due to oxidation) and freeze in ice cube trays, then store the fruit cubes in a bag in the freezer. I am more inclined to do this with apples and pears in winter and spring, when they are not really in season anymore, to preserve for summer.

WINTER GREENS

Bursting with flavor, winter greens are superfoods in their own right!

Celery   Celery is well known to be excellent for digestion. This is due to its nonstarch polysaccharide apiuman, which exerts an anti-inflammatory effect on the walls of the digestive tract, and its phthalides, which do the same, in addition to giving celery its characteristic scent and diuretic properties. Celery is a good source of vitamin K and folate, and is particularly rich in over a dozen phenolic antioxidants such as anti-inflammatory luteolin and blood vessel–protective kaempferol.

Collards   Collards have the highest cholesterol-lowering ability and the highest folate level of all the vegetables in the brassica family. Like other brassicas, collards assist with liver detoxification, because high levels of antioxidants facilitate phase I detox, and sulphur-containing nutrients support phase II detox. Rich in vitamins A, C, and folate, as well as manganese, and calcium, collards are also a good source of tryptophan and choline, which are important for mood.

Fennel   This anise-scented and -flavored vegetable is either loved or hated. Its characteristic scent of fennel comes from its volatile oil anethole, which is anti-inflammatory, anticancer, antifungal, and anti-bacterial! Fennel is a good source of manganese and vitamins C, K, and folate. Moreover, it is rich in the antioxidant flavonoid rutin, which helps to intensify the activity of vitamin C and strengthen capillaries, so it's good for people who bruise easily.

Kale　In addition to cancer protection for the breast, colon, and prostate common to brassicas, kale also protects against bladder and ovarian cancer. Rich in glucosinolates, carotenoid and chlorophyll pigments (and anthocyanins in red/purple kale varieties), and with over 45 flavonoids such as kaempferol and quercetin, kale's anti-inflammatory antioxidant power is substantial. Compared to all other brassicas, kale's level of vitamin K is at least double, making it a powerhouse for prevention of diseases such as diabetes, Alzheimer's, and arthritis. Kale is also very rich in vitamin A and a great source of vitamin C, manganese, copper, tryptophan, calcium, vitamin B6, and potassium.

Spinach　Like kale, spinach is a treasure trove of nutrition! Part of the chenopod family alongside beets, chard, and quinoa, spinach is second only to kale in its vitamin K content and is also an excellent source of vitamins A, C, E, B2, and B6, and folate, manganese, magnesium, iron, calcium, potassium, and tryptophan. Spinach is, unsurprisingly, rich in anti-inflammatory carotenoids and flavonoids, and in particular has an abundant carotenoid group called epoxyxanthophylls, which are thought to be the reason spinach has shown the best protection by a leafy green against prostate cancer, even more so than brassicas such as kale. Spinach also contains glycoglycerolipids, which are involved in photosynthesis and help protect against inflammation to the digestive tract.

THE WINTER GARDEN

In milder climates where it doesn't snow in winter, a lovely harvest of Asian greens, cabbage, kale, radishes, and spinach can be on offer with the efforts of planting in autumn. Continual planting of the quicker-growing greens such as bok choy, radishes, and spinach will ensure an ongoing supply over winter and into spring. If growing greens in your garden in winter is too difficult due to harsher climates, try growing sprouts and microgreens indoors (see page 33).

In late winter, celery can be planted, as can peas and lettuce varieties. To protect from frosts, create a warmer microclimate by covering plants overnight or planting them in a greenhouse. Try growing in pots and then move them to the sunniest areas of your garden, and consider planting near a sun-exposed brick wall for some radiant heat.

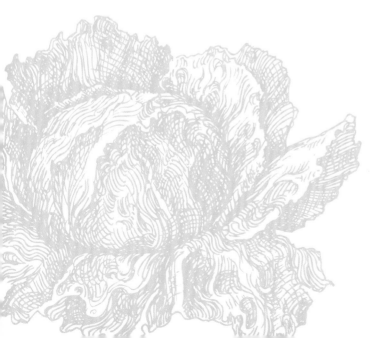

Lemon Liver Cleanser

Parsley and lemons are abundant in winter, and for a very good reason! Rich in immune-boosting vitamin C and detoxifying nutrients, this smoothie is perfect for getting a sluggish winter liver back in tip-top shape.

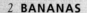

2 **BANANAS**

zest of 1 **LEMON**

flesh of 2 **LEMONS**, *seeded*

1½ cups **WATER**

1 to 2 handfuls of **PARSLEY**

AGAVE SYRUP OR HONEY, *to taste*

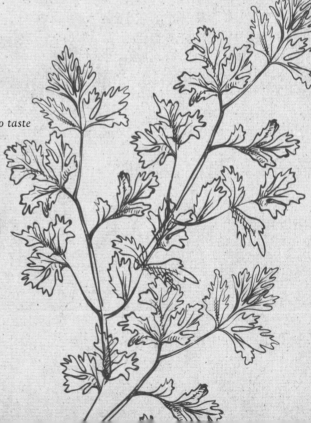

Waldorf Wonder

Inspired by the humble Waldorf salad, created at the Waldorf Hotel in New York City in the late 1800s, this green smoothie is fiber rich, tasty, and filling!

1 **APPLE**

1 **BANANA**

1 **CELERY RIB**

1 cup **WATER**

6 **WALNUT HALVES**

½ cup **ICE CUBES**

2 to 3 **MEDJOOL DATES**

handful of pale **CELERY LEAVES**

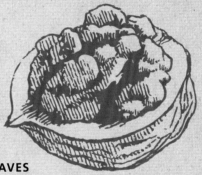

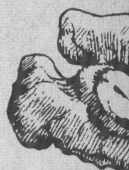

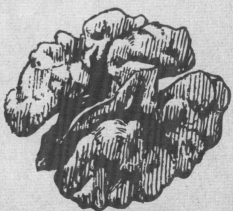

Heart Starter

Both tangelos and fennel are rich in heart-friendly potassium and a range of B vitamins, and together they taste simply sensational! To thicken the smoothie, use another cardiovascular booster, omega-laden chia seeds, which absorb ten times their size in liquid!

4 **TANGELOS**, *peeled*

1 cup **FENNEL JUICE**

1 to 2 tablespoons **CHIA SEEDS**

1 to 2 handfuls of **FENNEL TOPS**

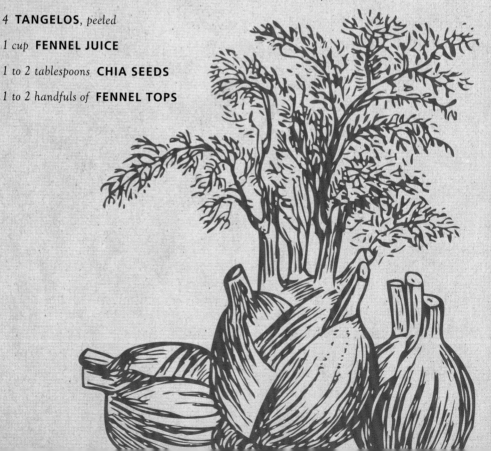

Kiwi Kooler

Considered a lost food from Incan times, tamarillos were reintroduced into New Zealand in the late 1800s and renamed using the Maori word *tama*, meaning leadership. They're not well known or widely available around the world so if you can find them, absolutely give them a try! Incredibly rich in vitamins, minerals, and antioxidants, this smoothie is a nutrient-dense crowd-pleaser!

flesh of 4 **TAMARILLOS**

1 frozen **BANANA**, sliced

¼ cup **RAISINS**, soaked in 1 cup water overnight

1 teaspoon **VANILLA EXTRACT**

1 cup **ALMOND MILK**

2 to 3 large leaves **SWISS CHARD**

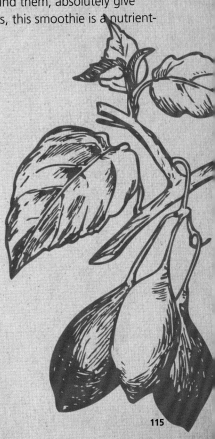

Green Machine

Love it or hate it, cilantro is like a multivitamin pill all wrapped up in one plant. With the sweet tang of pineapple, this green smoothie is the boost your body needs this winter!

1½ cups diced **PINEAPPLE**

1 **BANANA**

squeeze of **LIME OR LEMON JUICE**

1 cup **WATER**

1 to 2 handfuls of **CILANTRO**

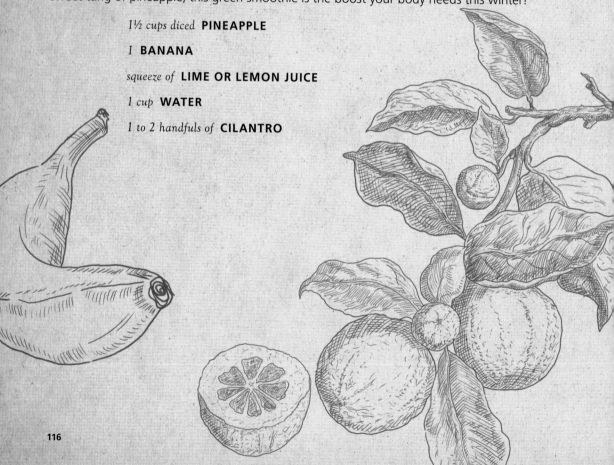

Bone Builder

With more vitamin C than oranges, the kiwifruit (or Chinese gooseberry), also has omega-3 fats in its seeds, as well as bone-health-promoting vitamin K and magnesium. With calcium-packed radish leaves, this smoothie is simply a bonanza for your bones!

2 **BANANAS**

1 **KIWIFRUIT**

1 **TANGELO OR ORANGE**, *peeled*

1½ *cups* **WATER**

1 to 2 handfuls of **RADISH TOPS**

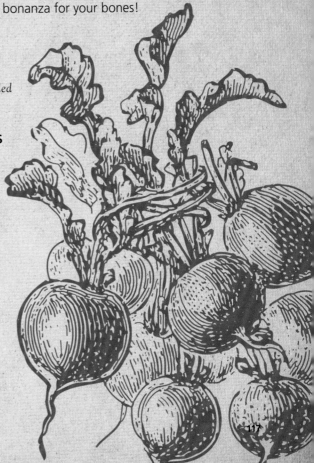

Mandarin Mania

Clementines and tangerines are well-known varieties of Mandarin oranges, and Mandarins like all citrus, are vitamin C rich and have a beautiful, distinct flavor. Of all citrus fruit, Mandarins have the highest levels of the antioxidant hesperidin, which works synergistically with vitamin C in the formation of collagen for skin and soft tissue healing.

2 cups peeled and seeded **MANDARIN ORANGE SEGMENTS**

1 cup diced **PINEAPPLE**

1 cup **WATER**

small handful of **TURNIP GREENS**

small handful of **SPINACH**

Pink Panther

Closely resembling blood plasma, coconut water is full of electrolyte minerals, enzymes, and B vitamins. When coconut water is paired with antioxidant-packed pomegranate and pale napa cabbage leaves, the result is that this "green" smoothie is actually a smashing pink-colored drink. Thicken with chia seeds, if desired.

juice and flesh of 1 **COCONUT**

juice of 1 large **POMEGRANATE***

1 to 2 tablespoons **COCONUT SUGAR OR NECTAR**

1 cup **WATER**

3 to 4 **NAPA CABBAGE LEAVES**

1 to 2 tablespoons **CHIA SEEDS** *(optional)*

* *To juice pomegranates, peel and blend whole, then strain through a nut milk bag or cheesecloth.*

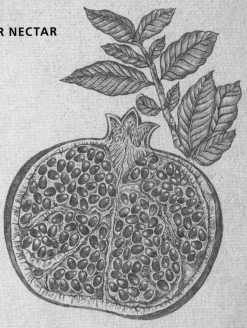

Creamy Pear Persuasion

The combination of beautiful winter pears and creamy seeds makes this a great alternative to banana-based smoothies. Rich in soluble fiber, pears are fantastic for blood sugar regulation and keeping *you* regular!

3 large ripe **PEARS**

2 to 3 tablespoons **HEMP OR SUNFLOWER SEEDS**

1½ cups **ALMOND MILK OR WATER**

1 to 2 (⅛-inch) slices **FRESH GINGER**

6 leaves **GREEN-STEM BOK CHOY**

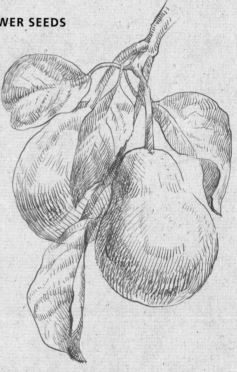

Mid-Winter's Warmth

This is the perfect concoction for a cold morning in the middle of winter when you need a kick of energy and a boost for your immune system. The ginger and spices are all antioxidant-rich additions to help keep the common cold far away.

2 **BANANAS**

1 *large* **PEAR**

½ *to 1 teaspoon* **GROUND CINNAMON**

pinch of **GROUND CLOVES**

¼ *teaspoon* **GROUND CARDAMOM**

2 *(⅛-inch) slices* **FRESH GINGER**

1 *teaspoon* **VANILLA EXTRACT**

1½ *cups* **ALMOND MILK**

handful of **KALE**

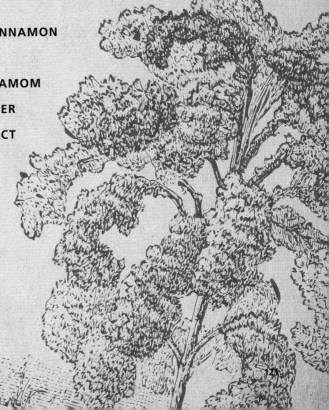

Turn Back the Clock

The key to longevity is to eat a diet rich in antioxidants, leafy greens, and B vitamins to keep disease-causing homocysteine amino acid low. High homocysteine promotes inflammation, which promotes aging. This anti-aging green smoothie will have you checking to see if those wrinkles are disappearing!

1 **APPLE**

¼ cup diced **BEETS**

½ small **AVOCADO**

½ cup **ICE**

1 cup **APPLE JUICE**

¼ cup dried **GOJI BERRIES**
(*soak overnight in the apple juice*)

6 to 8 **BEET GREENS WITH STEMS**

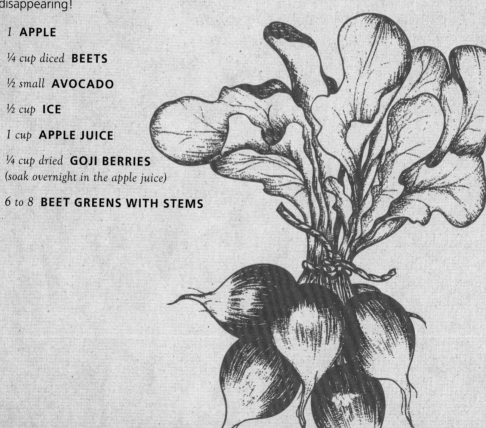

Alphabet Smoothie

With vitamin A from the grapefruit, vitamin B6 from the banana, vitamin C from the oranges, and vitamin E from the avocado, this smoothie covers your vitamin needs all in one happy place. For vitamin D, drink it in the sunshine!

1 large **PINK OR RED GRAPEFRUIT**, *seeded and peeled*

1 **BANANA**

½ **AVOCADO**

1½ cups **ORANGE JUICE**

2 handfuls of **SPINACH**

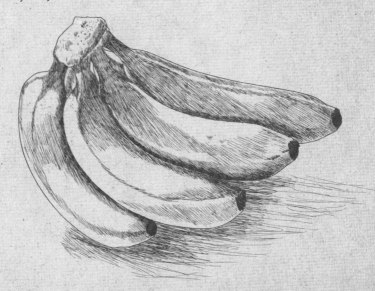

Savory Splendor

Rich and filling, this fragrant smoothie, with a hint of sweetness from the apple, is a delight at any time of day. As nutritional powerhouses, parsley and celeriac deliver bone-, blood-, and cell-building minerals in abundance.

1 cup diced **CELERIAC (CELERY ROOT)**

1 **GRANNY SMITH APPLE**

1½ cups **WATER**

⅓ cup **MACADAMIA NUTS**

½ cup **ICE CUBES**

small bunch of **PARSLEY**

pinch of **SALT AND PEPPER**

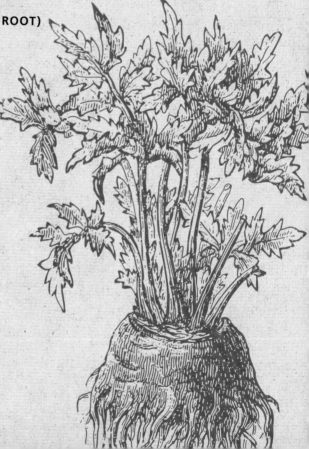

INDEX

All recipes are indexed, as are all *major* ingredients. Sweeteners, spices, optional ingredients, and small quantities of citrus are not indexed.

ARTWORK CREDITS

All images are from Shutterstock.com except where noted.

ABOUT THE AUTHOR

KRISTINE MILES is a health professional with over 17 years of experience. She is passionate about life-long learning, plant-based nutrition, and living a low-toxin lifestyle. Her mission is to promote health and well-being through empowering others to lead lives free of chemicals and full of real, delicious food. Kristine works as a physiotherapist in private practice and is a part-time cooking demonstrator, magazine contributor, and blogger at www.kristinemiles.com. Kristine's best-selling book *The Green Smoothie Bible* was released in February 2012. She is happily married and lives by the stunning surf coast of Phillip Island, Australia, with her husband and daughter.